Parkinson's Disease

AUTHORS

Paul J. Tuite, MD, is an associate professor of neurology and director of the Movement Disorders Program at the University of Minnesota. He received his medical degree from Indiana University and completed his neurology residency at McGill University. Additional training included a postgraduate fellowship in clinical electromyography (EMG) at McGill University and a neurophysiology and movement disorders fellowship at the University of Toronto. Since his arrival at Minnesota in 1996, Dr. Tuite has conducted over 30 clinical trials for Parkinson's disease (PD). His primary areas of research have related to the use of magnetic resonance imaging (MRI) in PD as well as the assessment of movement in PD, with the goal of advancing movement-related physical therapies for patients.

Cathi A. Thomas, RN, MS, is an assistant clinical professor of neurology and is program director of the Parkinson's Disease and Movement Disorder Center at Boston University Medical Center. She is the coordinator of the American Parkinson Disease Association Information and Referral Center at Boston University Medical Center and is a member of the Parkinson Study Group. During the past 25 years Ms. Thomas has provided care to individuals with Parkinson's disease and their families. As a clinical nurse specialist in neurorehabilitation, she has developed programs to assess the impact of Parkinson's disease on a patient and family and to assist them in coping with this condition.

Laura F. Ruekert, PharmD, RPh, is an assistant professor of pharmacy practice at Butler University and a clinical pharmacy specialist in behavioral care at Community North Hospital in Indianapolis, Indiana. She is director of a newly established Geriatric Psychiatry-Neurology Residency for Pharmacists. As well, she lectures on a variety of neurological and psychiatric topics to patients and pharmacy and nursing students, as well as internal medicine residents. Her clinical practice is as leader of an interdisciplinary team to provide excellent patient care, evaluate pharmacotherapy, and monitor patient outcomes. She completed an American Society of Health System Pharmacists (ASHP)–accredited Pharmacy Practice Residency with a focus in psychiatry at the University of Minnesota Medical Center.

Hubert H. Fernandez, MD, is associate professor of neurology and director of Clinical Trials for Movement Disorders, co-director of the Movement Disorders Program, and program director of the Neurology Residency Training Program and the Movement Disorders Fellowship Training Program, all at the University of Florida. He received his medical degree in the Philippines, and completed his neurology residency at Boston University and a postgraduate fellowship in movement disorders at Brown University. He is a Fellow of the American Academy of Neurology (also Executive Board Member of its Movement Disorders Section) and an active member of several professional societies, including the Movement Disorders Society, where he chaired the Task Force on Parkinson Psychosis Scales, and the Florida Society of Neurology, where he is currently the president-elect. He has authored over

over 100 peer-reviewed clinical publications on PD and other movement disorders. He is currently the medical editor of the Movement Disorders Society Web Site (www.movementdisroders.org).

CONTRIBUTOR

Narayan Kissoon, BS, is a medical student at the University of Minnesota Medical School.

Parkinson's Disease

A Guide to Patient Care

PAUL J. TUITE, MD
CATHI A. THOMAS, RN, MS
LAURA F. RUEKERT, PharmD, RPH
HUBERT H. FERNANDEZ, MD

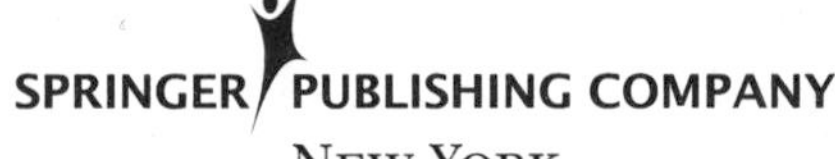

NEW YORK

Springer Publishing Company, LLC
11 West 42nd Street
New York, NY 10036
www.springerpub.com

Acquisitions Editor: Allan Graubard
Production Editor: Julia Rosen
Cover design: Mimi Flow
Composition: Apex CoVantage

09 10 11 12/ 5 4 3 2 1

Library of Congress Cataloging-in-Publication Data

Parkinson's disease : a guide to patient care / Paul Tuite … [et al.].
p. ; cm.
Includes bibliographical references and index.
ISBN 978-0-8261-2268-1 (alk. paper)
1. Parkinson's disease—Patients—Care—Handbooks, manuals, etc. I. Tuite, Paul.
[DNLM: 1. Parkinson Disease—theraphy—Handbooks. 2. Parkinson Disease—complications—Handbooks. 3. Parkinson Disease—diagnosis—Handbooks.
WL 39 P247 2009]
RC382.P247 2009
616.8'33—dc22 2008046032

Printed in the United States of America by Bang Printing.

This book is dedicated to people with Parkinson's disease along with their families and friends. May this reference ease the process of dealing with the challenges PD brings.

We also would like to dedicate this book to our parents, siblings, spouses, and children, who have helped make us whole.

P.J.T.

C.A.T.

L.F.R.

H.H.F.

Contents

Preface

We have heard time and again of the extraordinary difference a health care professional can make in the quality of life of a person and family living with Parkinson's disease. Witness the *nurse* who is working in an adult day center and makes the specific effort to provide the Parkinson patient's medication on time; or the *physical therapist* who designs an exercise plan that the patient can self-adapt long after services have ended. It may be the *physician* who learns of new clinical trial opportunities and takes the time to call and share this information with the Parkinson patient, or the *psychologist* who avoids added medications by training a patient to use relaxation therapy to relieve his or her anxiety.

Living with Parkinson's disease presents numerous challenges to our patients and families. The disease is an unavoidable intrusion into the life of not only the patient but also the patient's spouse, children, parents, and social networks.

Most individuals are diagnosed in the fifth and sixth decade—during the prime of their life—and up to 10% of patients receive their diagnosis before the age of 40. This moment of diagnosis often occurs in the midst of the challenges of raising children and establishing a career—almost certainly before most patients have had the chance to garner the financial resources necessary to live with a chronic illness. The disease itself is complex, with both motor and nonmotor symptoms. Although advances in medical and surgical therapies have greatly improved patients' function and quality of life, the medication management of PD necessitates careful and frequent adjustments, requiring a dynamic balance between the drug's benefit and the risk of adverse effects.

As *health care professionals* we need to assist our patients in meeting these complex and interwoven challenges. This might include spending hours during an office visit programming a DBS stimulator to obtain the best possible outcome, or answering an end-of-the-day call to counsel an anxious patient who is about to lose a job owing to increasing disability.

Meeting these challenges requires a sophisticated understanding of the disease process and available therapies, with an appreciation that each patient's experience with PD is unique and responds best to an individualized plan of care.

This book was written to provide information to health care professionals involved in the many aspects of the care of PD patients and their families in all health care settings. With this in mind, we have created a practical compendium on management issues related to PD—a framework that one can individualize for their specific health care setting. With the increasing numbers of patients with PD—numbers that are expected to double by 2030—there is an increasing need for help with troubleshooting patient issues. It is designed as a quick reference acknowledging that our current health care environment has mandated that exceptional care be provided with not enough time or resources.

This book is divided into four main parts: *problems, evaluation, treatment,* and the *appendices.* The first section on *problems* is arranged alphabetically so that the provider does not need to classify what organ system a symptom or problem belongs to. We realize that problems can overlap and are sometimes vague, such as fatigue, pain, and weight loss, and are difficult to conveniently categorize. The second section is on *evaluation,* since, not uncommonly, Parkinson patients require numerous evaluations throughout the duration of their illness such as genetic testing, brain imaging, speech and swallowing evaluation, and so forth. The third section deals with *treatment.* Here we divided the module into pharmacological and nonpharmacological sections. The medications are grouped according to their use in Parkinson's disease. Equally important are the nonpharmacological treatments such as nutritional, physical, occupational, sleep, and speech therapy, and of course, deep brain stimulation surgery. We end the book with *appendices* of medication handouts, available resources list, and compilation of scales used in Parkinson's disease, that will help the health care professional in delivering the best possible care to the Parkinson patient.

We hope you will benefit from the wisdom we have gained from our highly motivated and resilient patients and families. We do not have all of the answers and certainly welcome ideas and suggestions from you.

Paul J. Tuite
Cathi Ann Thomas
Laura F. Ruekert
Hubert H. Fernandez

Acknowledgments

The authors would like to thank the following individuals for their guidance, careful review, and generous support during the writing of this book: Donna Diaz, RN, MS; Terry Ellis, PhD, RPT, NCS; Tim Ferry; Joseph Furtado, RN, MS; Tami Rork, MS, RPT; and Marie Saint Hilaire, MD, FRCPC. We would also like to acknowledge the University of Minnesota Medical Foundation for its generous support.

Problems

SECTION I

ANXIETY

Anxiety is a common yet undertreated symptom of Parkinson's disease (PD) characterized by nervousness, fear, or intense worry. Symptoms can range from an uneasy feeling that something will go wrong to a severe panic attack. In PD anxiety occurs in up to 40% of individuals and may accompany depression. It can present itself in three ways:

1. It can be one of the initial symptoms of the disease and may precede motor difficulties by years. Symptoms of generalized anxiety disorder may fluctuate a little but are often pervasive in nature unless treated. They are usually not related to the use of Parkinson medications.
2. Individuals who have fluctuations in motor symptoms often have heightened anxiety as their medications begin to wear off. The symptoms of anxiety may lessen with the initiation or an increase in the dose of anti-Parkinson medications.
3. Some patients experience *internal tremor*. They feel tremulous inside but the tremor is not apparent externally. Internal tremors are often associated with anxiety.

Assessment

Routinely screen for anxiety. The Beck Anxiety Instrument (BAI) is a self-administered screening tool used clinically to discriminate anxiety from depression.

Assess anxiety as it relates to Parkinson symptoms and/or treatments.

- When does it occur?
- How long does it last?
- What does the patient experience?
- Is there a relationship between the anxiety and medication response, that is, wearing off or "off" periods (when medication effect has completely diminished)?

Careful medical history and a physical exam are done to rule out other causes of anxiety or anxiety disorders and differentiate from other PD symptoms including internal tremor or restless leg syndrome. Pulse, blood pressure, and respiratory rate often increase with anxiety. Blood tests (CBC, thyroid function tests) as well as an electrocardiogram (ECG) may be done to look for treatable conditions causing anxiety. Referral to a mental health care professional can be useful for assessment and treatment.

Nonpharmacological Management

- Provide patient/family education on the signs and symptoms of anxiety, potential triggers of anxiety, and lifestyle changes that decrease anxiety.
- Practice good sleep hygiene.
- Exercise regularly.
- Limit caffeine and alcohol.
- Avoid nicotine or other recreational drugs.
- Share information on the use of relaxation techniques including guided imagery, massage, yoga, tai chi, or meditation.
- Provide referral for biofeedback, administered by a certified health care professional.
- Provide referral for psychological counseling.

Pharmacological Management

Use of Parkinson's Disease Medications

- If anxiety or a panic attack appears during wearing-off spells, then anxiety may respond to optimization of Parkinson's disease medications. The anxiety may improve in parallel to the effects on tremor, gait, and slowness. Carbidopa/levodopa and/or dopamine agonists may be useful.

Use of Antianxiety Medications

- These medications have a calming effect and belong to a class of medications called anxiolytics. These drugs if used chronically can cause tolerance, which requires gradually increasing doses to get a desired effect. A withdrawal condition can occur, including seizures if the drugs are discontinued abruptly. A common side effect of these medications is sleepiness, so extreme caution should be used if operating heavy machinery (e.g., driving a car) while under treatment with these medications. Most commonly within this group of medications are benzodiazepines, which share a similar chemical structure. Commonly prescribed antianxiety medications include Lorazepam (Ativan®) and Clonazepam (Klonopin®). This class of drugs is also helpful for internal tremors as well as visible tremors.

Use of Antidepressant Medications

- The selective serotonin reuptake inhibitors (SSRIs), for example, paroxetine and sertraline, have become the most commonly employed medication treatment of depression and have been shown to have an effect on anxiety. As with all medications, starting with a low dose and increasing after one or two weeks to a desired dose is typical. Concern has been raised about adverse interaction between SSRIs and selegiline or rasagaline. Adverse interaction is rare. Most SSRIs at their typical dose should not have it, but some do, and a consultation with a physician or pharmacist will help clarify this. Patients should be instructed to contact the physician or a health care provider immediately if they present with signs of a serotonin syndrome, including tachycardia, diaphoresis, myoclonic twitching, hypertension, and hyperthermia.

Patient/Family Educational Resources

Friedman, J. H. (2008). *Making the connection between brain and behavior: Coping with Parkinson's disease.* New York: Demos Health.

APATHY

The motor deficits seen in Parkinson's disease patients as well as nonmotor manifestations including depression and fatigue can lead to a decrease in motivation or lack of interest in normal life activities. However, some individuals experience what is defined as *apathy*. This affective disorder presents as a flat mood, indifference, decreased concern, and lack of drive in persons with PD. Apathy can occur alone or in conjunction with many conditions, particularly psychiatric disturbances.

A hallmark of apathy is that it is not noticeable or of concern to the persons experiencing it. However, it can be extremely distressing to family members as well as other social contacts. In addition, those with apathy are less inclined to properly care for themselves because they simply are not motivated. This self-care deficit can affect the overall sense of well-being and health status of individuals.

It should be noted that many patients with PD remain highly optimistic and very active throughout the course of their illness. Additional studies are needed to better understand why some individuals experience apathy and others do not.

Assessment

- Medical history and physical examination to identify signs and symptoms of apathy are necessary. Individuals with apathy will rarely bring to the attention of health care providers that they are apathetic. Family members will provide information and often will voluntarily express their concerns.
- Referral to a neuropsychologist and/or psychiatrist is useful to differentiate from the diagnosis of depression.
- The Neuropsychiatric Inventory Questionnaire (NPI-Q) addresses apathy with the following item. This is administered to spouses or other family caregivers:

Apathy or Indifference: Does the patient seem less interested in his or her usual activities and in the activities and plans of others?

Nonpharmacological Management

- Provide support to families and/or caregivers by recognizing the problem. Discuss the fact that the apathetic experience is usually not bothersome to the patient and, understandably, is more bothersome to family members.
- Refer caregivers to counseling or a support group to assist in dealing with patient apathy.
- Family members and health care providers should assess whether apathy is interfering with a patient's ability to provide self-care.
- Family members should identify and assist patients in participating in activities that are still enjoyable.

Pharmacological Management

- There is no known pharmacological treatment for apathy.
- A trial of antidepressant medications may be useful in the event there is this psychiatric comorbidity.

CAREGIVER ROLE STRAIN

As a health care professional, providing comprehensive care for an individual with Parkinson's disease should include a thorough assessment of the person's caregiver support system. This can include a spouse or significant other, often the primary caregiver, as well as children and parents. Chronic illness is a family experience. The complexity of PD presents numerous stressors not only on the patient but also the family, most often the primary caregiver. This can lead to caregiver stress and oftentimes burnout.

Assessment of family coping strategies should take place at the time of diagnosis and continue throughout the course of the person's illness. Evidence suggests that certain risk factors including the health of the family caregiver, presence of depression, quality of relationships among family members, and decreased optimism increase the likelihood of caregiver strain. Advancing disability and cognitive impairment place additional burdens on family caregivers.

Patients, family members, and caregivers benefit from appropriate information throughout the trajectory of the illness. Information on the disease process including signs and symptoms, prognosis, and available treatments allows one to better anticipate care needs and plan for the present and future.

Assessment

Assessment of the patient and family in the context of caregiving can be performed by all members of the health care team. Information important in determining the presence or risk of caregiver strain includes:

- Physical and psychosocial health status of caregiver
- Physical and psychosocial health status of person with PD
- Familial roles and responsibilities
- Ability to provide care
- Financial resources
- Social support network

Management

- Provide an opportunity to discuss the role of caring for the individual with PD with both the patient and family. Discussion should not only address the health and wellness concerns of the patient but also the caregiver.
- Share strategies with both the patient and caregiver to improve health and wellness, including the importance of good nutrition, regular physical activity, adequate rest and sleep, stress reduction, and maintaining social connections.
- Provide information and referrals to home health care agencies, adult day programs, respite care, assisted living, and long-term care as appropriate.
- Refer to a mental health provider including a licensed social worker or psychologist to provide individual or family counseling and support.
- Refer patient and/or family to Parkinson's disease and caregiver support groups.

Resources for Caregivers

- National Alliance for Caregiving
  4720 Montgomery Lane
  5th floor
  Bethesda, MD 20814
  www.caregiving.org
- National Family Caregivers Association
  10400 Connecticut Avenue, Suite 500
  Kensington, MD 20895-3944
  800-896-3650
  www.familycaregiver.org
- Well Spouse Association
  63 West Main Street, Suite H
  Freehold, NJ 07728
  800-838-0879
  www.wellspouse.org
- Family Caregiver Alliance
  180 Montgomery Street, Suite 1100
  San Francisco, CA 94104
  800-445-8106
  www.caregiver.org
- Children of Aging Parents
  P.O. Box 167
  Richboro, PA 18954
  800-227-7294
  www.caps4caregivers.org

COMPULSIVE BEHAVIORS

Individuals with Parkinson's disease may exhibit compulsive behaviors (often but not exclusively related to levodopa) or impulse control disorders (frequently associated with dopamine agonists). Individuals who have undergone deep brain stimulation (DBS) are also at risk. Examples of *impulsive behaviors* include obsessions with gambling, shopping, eating, or sex. Often reported by spouses is an increased interest by the person with PD to have sex or desire to watch pornography. These behaviors are rare but present significant psychosocial concerns for a patient and family. Examples of *compulsive behaviors* include the need for more and

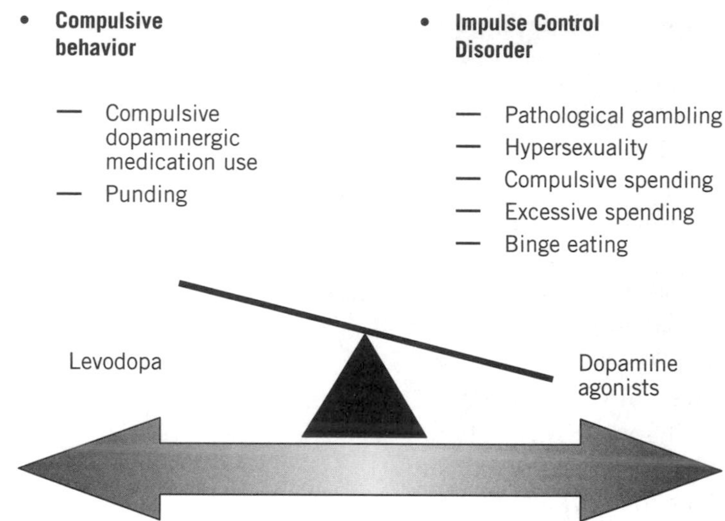

Figure 1.1 Compulsive and impulsive disorders in PD.

more levodopa, or preoccupation with performing certain activities over and over such as manipulating mechanical objects, weeding, sorting, collecting, and so forth (often referred to as *punding*). See Figure 1.1.

The cause is not fully understood but it is known that dopamine affects the brain's pleasure and reward centers. Studies are ongoing with dopamine agonists that stimulate dopamine receptors, particularly D3, located in the limbic system. It remains unclear if there is a preexisting so-called addictive personality or a tendency for compulsions that puts certain individuals with Parkinson's disease at risk. However, it can occur in patients with no history of addictive behavior. In general, levodopa has been implicated in compulsive behaviors and dopamine agonists have been associated with impulsive behaviors but there is significant overlap in these conditions.

Assessment

- Obtain a history of compulsive disorders or addictions before the initiation of drug therapy.
- Routinely inquire about the side effect of compulsive behaviors during treatment.
- Use the modified Minnesota Impulsive Disorders Interview (MIDI) to establish a baseline and for ongoing assessment.

Pharmacological Management

Consultation with neurologist/health care provider managing Parkinson's disease medications:

- Reduce or discontinue dopamine agonists or other PD meds.
- Manage PD symptoms if necessary with carbidopa/levodopa alone.
- Assess need for antipsychotic medication.
- Assess need for selective serotonin reuptake inhibitors (SSRIs).

Nonpharmacological Management

- Help the patient and family to understand what a compulsive behavior is and how and when to report these behaviors to a health care provider.
- Provide a referral to a psychiatrist and/or psychologist to assist the patient and family with problem recognition, ongoing treatment, and psychosocial support.

CONSTIPATION

Constipation is common in Parkinson's disease. Almost all individuals report a change in bowel habits, often before a diagnosis of PD is made. Patients will describe a change in routine that may include one or more of the following: a decrease in number of stools per week, change in consistency and size of stool, the presence of straining, the feeling of being bloated, and abdominal fullness or discomfort. Constipation can be intermittent or for some chronic and persistent. It can become all-consuming, leading to increased frustration for both the patient and family.

Constipation and other changes in bowel habits should always be assessed for relationship to other conditions or treatments. Complications include loss of appetite, incontinence, nausea and vomiting, impaction, fissures, rectal prolapse, hemorrhoids, syncope, and bowel obstruction. Bowel obstruction can be life-threatening and requires immediate attention.

A change in the autonomic nervous system in PD causes slowing of gastric and bowel motility, resulting in constipation. In addition, medications used to treat PD, including levodopa, anticholinergics, dopamine agonists, MAO-inhibitors, and amantadine are contributors. Finally, lifestyle factors including lack of exercise, poor dietary habits, and a decreased ability to toilet increase the risk of constipation.

Assessment

- Patient history must be taken.
- For severe constipation, physical examination by the primary care provider/gastrointestinal (GI) specialist will include evaluation of physical function, abdominal assessment, a rectal examination, and a neurological evaluation of the anal reflex. In addition, laboratory and/or radiographic tests may be ordered.
- Colorectal cancer screening by primary care provider/GI specialist including annual fecal occult blood tests and age-appropriate colonoscopy is necessary.

Management

Constipation is managed using a stepwise approach. It may take several weeks for a person with PD to establish normal bowel patterns. Constipation is managed in a stepwise approach described by Folden (2002), which is an adaptation of the approach described by Sandburg, McGuire, and Lee (1996).

Step 1—Lifestyle Changes

- *Increase Exercise and Activity.* Walking, lower trunk rotation, and stationary bicycling enhance bowel function. Individuals with PD should perform exercise regularly. Exercise is easier to perform in the "on" state, when medications are in full effect.
- *Change Dietary Habits.* Increase dietary fiber. Meals should include fruits, vegetables, and whole grain selections. A nutritional consultation is useful.
- *Try "Power Pudding."* Mix together (may use a blender or spoon) a proportion of prune juice (or pitted prunes), and processed bran and applesauce such that the viscosity should be a thickened paste. Take a tablespoon of mixture with water daily. Refrigerate the remainder of the mixture.
- *Increase Fluid Intake.* Drink 6–8 glasses of liquid per day. Caffeine and alcoholic beverages should be avoided.

- *Establish a Regular Toileting Regime.* Identify a consistent time for a bowel movement, usually within 30 minutes of the morning meal. Do not avoid the urge to move bowels. The person should be in an upright position. Individuals with PD have difficulty expelling feces and may benefit from placing their feet on a footstool in front of the toilet.
- If no bowel movement occurs after three days, proceed to step 2 and/or step 3.

Step 2—Use of Bulk-Forming Agents

- These include methylcellulose (Citrucel®), psyllium (Metamucil®), dietary bran, and polycarbophil (FiberCon®). These over-the-counter medications are used daily and should be taken with a full glass of water. Good hydration is important for effectiveness.

Step 3—Use of Stool Softeners

- Softeners moisten and soften hard dry stool and are used daily as needed.
- Common agents include docusate sodium (Colace®) and lubiprostone (Amitiza®).
- If constipation continues after treatment with steps 1, 2, and 3, add step 4.

Step 4—Use of Osmotic Laxatives

- Osmotive laxative agents include saline laxatives (milk of magnesia) and hyperosmotic agents (lactulose, sorbitol, MiraLax®, and glycerin suppository). These agents stimulate intestinal motility. They should be used sparingly because they can be habit-forming.

Step 5—Stimulant Agents

- Agents include bisocodyl, cascara sagrada, and senna. These should be used only for short-term management of constipation because they chemically irritate the bowel.

Step 6—Suppository/Enemas

- The final step in treating constipation is the use of suppositories (glycerin, bisacodyl [Dulcolax]®) or enemas (Fleets®). Glycerin suppositories are the mildest and should be tried first.

References

Folden, S. L. (2002). Practice guidelines for the management of constipation in adults. *Rehabilitation Nursing, 27*(5), 169–175.

Sandburg, A. L., McGuire, T. M., & Lee, T. (1996). Stepping out of constipation: An educational campaign. *Australian Journal of Hospital Pharmacy, 26,* 350–355.

DEPRESSION

Depression is characterized by feelings of sadness, worthlessness, fatigue, and a decreased interest in activities, usually for a period greater than 1–2 weeks. Most people feel this way at one time or another for short periods of time, but true clinical depression occurs when these feelings are present for an extended time and interfere with everyday life. Depression occurs in about 40%–70% of people with PD and is often accompanied by anxiety. These nonmotor symptoms can appear years before the motor features of PD. Depression is not always recognized by either the patient or the health care provider, and even when recognized, it is often undertreated.

Depression may be caused, in part, by a loss of nerve cells other than dopaminergic cells, which produce norepinephrine or serotonin. It can also be reactive, that is, based on something that is happening in a person's life, such as increased stress at work or the appearance of a new symptom. In PD it is probably caused by a combination of chemical changes in the brain as well as experiences related to having a chronic health condition. Antidepressant therapy is usually very effective; however, studies are needed to determine the best pharmacological and nonpharmacological treatment approaches.

Assessment

Assessment of depression in PD is complex. Many of the signs we use to identify depression are effects of Parkinson's itself and do not always indicate a change in mood. For example, decreased facial expression in PD, slowness in movement and thinking, irregular sleep patterns, and other such symptoms can be misinterpreted as sadness or depression. Patients and families should always be asked about their mood during a health evaluation.

It is also important to distinguish between depression (a feeling of sadness; "feeling blue") and apathy (which is characterized by indifference or lack of interest in people, events, or surroundings). Apathy can accompany depression but can also occur in isolation. It is important to differentiate between the two conditions because depression often responds to antidepressant medications, while there is no known pharmacological treatment for apathy.

A complete medical history, family history, review of medications, and a physical exam are all important. As in other populations, it is important to rule out secondary causes of depression before proceeding to pharmacological treatments. This workup may include a complete blood count, liver function tests, serum testosterone levels, and thyroid function tests. It is important to review current medications, as many drugs can have depressive side effects. A unique point to pursue with the PD patient is whether the depressive symptoms relate to motor fluctuations or the timing of PD medications. Depressive symptoms may be a nonmotor manifestation of an "off" state in some patients and may be improved by smoothing out these fluctuations.

The Beck Depression Scale, the Geriatric Depression Scale, and the Hamilton Depression Scale have been used in clinical trials in PD. To date there is not a scale specific to PD.

Assessment by a mental health care professional is recommended for individuals with moderate to severe depression.

Depression in the patient often affects the entire family unit. It is important to assess the impact depression has on a spouse, on children, or on others in the patient's social network.

Nonpharmacological Management

- Patients and families should be informed on how to recognize potential signs of depression including change in mood, loss of interest in usual activities, overwhelming feelings of guilt, sleep disturbance (both insomnia and hypersomnolence), decrease in appetite, weight loss, anxiety, decreased feelings of self-worth, feelings of incapacity, fatigue, decrease in libido, and suicidal ideations (which are rare in PD).
- Patients and families should be told that being apathetic does not necessarily mean that a Parkinson patient is depressed. Lack of interest in surroundings or unwillingness to participate or engage in activities may not necessarily reflect sadness or lack of caring.
- Provide a referral to a mental health professional.

- Psychological or talk therapy may be used to treat depression and anxiety. One form of therapy, cognitive behavioral therapy, helps individuals alter their coping methods by changing the way they think about their condition and life circumstances. Meeting with mental health professionals can assist patients to learn techniques to increase their resilience and ability to cope.
- Psychotherapy can be used to treat symptoms by attempting to identify the cause of the problem. Psychotherapy is an individualized and interactive process that can be applied during short and long periods of time.
- Spouses and other family members may benefit from a referral to a mental health professional and caregiver support group to better cope with their loved one's depression.

Pharmacological Management

Use of Antidepressant Medications

- The selective serotonin reuptake inhibitors (SSRIs), such as paroxetine (Paxil®) and sertraline (Zoloft®), have become the most commonly employed medications for depression and have been shown to have an effect on anxiety. Fluoxetine (Prozac®) may increase physiologic tremor.
- Other medications used to treat depression in PD include bupropion (Wellbutrin®), venlafaxine (Effexor®), mirtazapine (Remeron®), and tricyclic antidepressants (TCAs) such as amitriptyline, doxepin, and imipramine. However, TCAs are now less commonly used to treat depression in the PD population.
- As with all antidepressants, one should begin with the lowest dose and increase the dosage after 1–2 weeks until the desired dose has been reached.

Concern has also been raised about adverse interaction between SSRIs and the MAO-B inhibitors selegiline and rasagaline. An adverse interaction is rare. Most SSRIs at their typical dose should not have this interaction. Patients should be instructed to contact their physician or a health care provider immediately if they present with possible signs of a "serotonin syndrome" including: tachycardia, diaphoresis, myoclonic twitching, hypertension, and hyperthermia.

Adjusting Anti-PD Medications

Sometimes depression is a manifestation of *wearing off*, when the effects of the PD medication start to decline. Often, wearing off is manifested by increased tremor, stiffness, and slowness, but it can also be manifested by depression, slowed thinking, fatigue, anxiety, or panic attacks. When wearing off occurs, it is best treated by augmenting or adjusting the anti-PD medications, for example, by increasing the frequency of dosing, or adding a "levodopa extender" such as entacapone.

DROOLING

Sialorrhea is the inability to control saliva in the oropharynx. This symptom affects up to 70% of individuals with PD. Some people may report a slight excess of saliva, often noted when they wake up to a wet pillow. Others experience marked drooling requiring constant use of tissues or a towel. Patients and families often express embarrassment, resulting in a decrease in socialization and quality of life. In addition, a buildup of saliva in the mouth may increase the risk of aspiration pneumonia.

The cause of drooling in PD is not fully understood but is thought to be related to reduced movement of the swallowing musculature, which results in less swallowing. This decrease in spontaneous or reflexive swallowing results in an excess of saliva in the mouth. A tendency to have lips open and/or lean forward increases the amount of saliva that leaves the mouth.

Assessment

The presence of drooling is noted by observation, as well as being reported by the patient and/or family. It may be useful to use the Unified Parkinson's Disease Rating Scale (UPDRS) item, Salivation, to rate drooling.

1. Normal
2. Slight but definite excess of saliva in mouth; may have nighttime drooling
3. Moderately excessive saliva; may have minimal drooling
4. Marked excess saliva with some drooling
5. Marked drooling, requires constant tissue or handkerchief

Nonpharmacological Management

- Provide a referral to a speech and language pathologist.
- Remind the patient to chew food slowly and carefully, swallowing frequently.
- Use (sugar-free) chewing gum or suck on hard candy (lozenges) to increase the swallowing reflex.
- Sometimes carrying a handkerchief or small towel at all times is the best strategy.

Pharmacological Management

- Anticholinergics such as Atropine or Robinul® may be prescribed to decrease drooling but often have side effects including confusion, hallucinations, urinary retention, and constipation.
- Certain antidepressants with anticholinergic effects (such as nortriptyline) for depression may also incidentally reduce drooling.
- Botulinum toxin (Botox® or Myobloc®) injections into salivary (parotid and submandibular) glands may decrease drooling; these injections are expensive and need to be repeated every few months.

Special Considerations

- Carbidopa/levodopa and dopamine agonists may improve swallowing but typically do not decrease drooling.
- In severe cases referral to an oral surgeon to explore removal of salivary glands may be indicated.

DYSKINESIA

Dyskinesias are involuntary movements, often writhing or choreiform, and are dance-like in nature. They are one of the motor complications of long-term levodopa therapy. However, dyskinesia can certainly appear earlier with the use of dopaminergic medications. They typically occur during the peak effectiveness of a dose of levodopa (termed peak dose dyskinesias) but can also take place at the beginning or at the end of a medication dose (termed diphasic dyskinesias). Dyskinesia may affect any part of the body including the extremities, trunk, neck, and facial muscles. Peak dose dyskinesias are often more severe on the side of the body most affected by PD. It should be noted that dyskinesia often increases during stress-related events, including a visit to the health care provider.

Patients often have difficulty self-recognizing mild and even moderate dyskinesia. Therefore, a family member is more likely to report this complication to the health care provider. Moderate to severe dyskinesia can be troublesome, especially when it affects gait, balance, and the ability to perform activities of daily living. Patients and caregivers may feel stigmatized when these involuntary movements are noticed by others.

Assessment

Careful history and observation are important in assessing dyskinesia. Information obtained should include the severity, relationship to medication dose, time of day, and activity level. The patient/care provider should be asked:

1 What proportion of the waking day is dyskinesia present?
2 How disabling is the dyskinesia?
3 Is there pain associated with the dyskinesia?

Patient diaries, completed at home, are useful tools to collect information. Dyskinesia rating scales exist but are used primarily in research settings.

Pharmacological Management

- Adjustment of levodopa: typically, this means reduction of dose or frequency.
- Adjustment of dopamine agonists: dose reduction is called for.
- Amantadine (Symmetrel®) provides consistent but only partial reduction of dyskinesia; dosing often begins with 100 mg twice a day (BID), then is increased to 100 mg three times a day (TID) as needed.

Nonpharmacological Management

- Patient/family education should include training on how to assess and document the presence of dyskinesia. Patient and family should be taught the difference between dyskinesia and tremor so that symptoms can be reported effectively.

- Patients and family members should be aware of the importance of maintaining a safe environment when dyskinesia is present, including ambulation safety, driving limitation, and modification of activities of daily living.
- Individuals with moderate to severe dyskinesia often have a significant decrease in dyskinesia following DBS surgery. Therefore, this intervention is often recommended if medication adjustment is not effective with this population.
- Psychological support should be provided to assist the patient/family in coping with the stigma associated with dyskinesia.

DYSTONIA

Dystonia as a symptom in PD is a sustained muscle contraction that is often described as a painful cramp. It can occur as part of the disease process or as a complication of dopaminergic medication.

For many individuals, particularly in young-onset PD, dystonia will be the first symptom reported to a physician. This may include flexion of the foot that worsens when walking, often accompanied by flexion of the toes (toe curling). It may also occur in an arm or the neck. Other dystonias in PD, sometimes observed later in the disease, include truncal dystonia, and blepharospasm (affecting the muscles of the eyelids).

Assessment

- Take a careful medical history, family history, and physical examination to determine the cause and type of dystonia. Dystonia is a disease entity within itself with many subtypes.
- Note the location of the dystonia, time of day of onset, degree of pain or discomfort, and any known tricks that are used by the patient to relieve dystonia.
- For individuals treated with levodopa and other PD medications, note any relationship to medication. Early morning dystonia occurs before a person takes a dose of levodopa. These cramps, usually in the legs or feet, can be painful and often wake the person up from a sound sleep.

Pharmacological Management

- Optimize PD medications in an attempt to decrease dystonia. This is trial and error depending on whether dystonia is related to too much dopamine, too little, or not at all.
- Botulinum toxin injections are used for certain types and locations of dystonia. This works by blocking the release of acetylcholine at the neuromuscular junction. It is administered by injection into the affected muscle. Electromyography guidance will be used when certain muscles are involved, especially those close to body organs, such as a lung. Although expensive, botulinum toxin treatment has significantly improved functional status and quality of life for many individuals. Thc duration of action is 3–4 months with patients receiving injections 3–4 times a year.

Nonpharmacological Management

- Use physical measures including massage, application of heat, and/or gentle stretching of the affected area.
- Advise the patient on proper shoe fitting. This is important for individuals who experience toe curling and foot dystonia.

FATIGUE

Fatigue is common in Parkinson's disease and can seem as much a state of mind as of body. It can occur in up to 40% of PD patients, and when felt is often one of the more disabling symptoms of PD. The feeling of fatigue is hard to describe and even more difficult to measure. Many symptoms of PD can cause a feeling of weariness and make it difficult for an individual to finish an activity. Fatigue can be related to slowness of movement, muscle stiffness, fluctuations in mobility, depression, and sleep disturbance. Fatigue related to PD is difficult to treat and only occasionally responds to anti-Parkinson medications.

Fatigue may be related to other health conditions including anemia, heart disease, low blood pressure, and diabetes, to name a few. In addition, medications that cause sedation, including sleep medications, antihypertensive drugs, allergy medications, medications for anxiety and depression, seizure medications, and muscle relaxants, all contribute to fatigue. Finally, individuals who are deconditioned from a lack of physical activity or are bored from a lack of meaningful stimuli are at risk for fatigue.

Therefore, fatigue can be an intrinsic feature of PD, a lack of medication, a result of deconditioning, a symptom of depression, a medication side effect, or a symptom of an unrelated medical condition. These possibilities will need to be sorted out in each PD patient.

Assessment

- Medical history and physical examination to identify the cause of fatigue
- An inventory of medications, including doses and timing, with a daily diary to determine if fatigue correlates with wearing-off periods
- Complete blood count
- Thyroid and chemistry panel
- Urinalysis if appropriate to look for a urinary tract infection
- Behavioral assessment for depression and apathy
- Primary care consultation to address the possibility of another condition causing fatigue

Nonpharmacological Management

Patient and family education includes the following information.

- Get adequate, regular, and consistent amounts of sleep each night.
- Eat a healthy, well-balanced diet.
- Eat a lot of fiber and drink plenty of fluids to avoid constipation.
- Exercise regularly including both aerobic and stretching exercises.
- Keep mentally active. Boredom often leads to fatigue.
- Use relaxation therapies including yoga or meditation.
- Maintain a reasonable work and personal schedule.
- Do more difficult tasks when movement is easier and medications are working well.
- Avoid alcohol, nicotine, and recreational drug use.

Pharmacological Management

- Although not well studied, modafinil, methylphenidate, and amantadine have been prescribed to treat fatigue.

- If fatigue is a manifestation of undermedication, increasing the medication doses may improve fatigue.
- If fatigue is a symptom of wearing off, adjusting medications (increasing the levodopa dosage, or adding an MAO-B inhibitor, COMT-inhibitor, or dopamine agonist) may relieve fatigue.
- If fatigue is part of depression, adding an antidepressant may help.

FREEZING

Freezing is the inability to initiate or continue a movement. It is usually a problem of gait in PD but can be observed with other motor tasks. Gait freezing strongly impacts a person's ability to move safely, with ease and confidence. For some, it is both disabling and frustrating and typically occurs later in the disease course. Gait freezing may indicate that a person is undermedicated, or can increase in incidence during periods of medication wearing off. However, it may not be related to Parkinson medication doses or "on" and "off" states at all.

The exact mechanism that causes freezing is unclear; it tends to occur during certain activities. People often report difficulty walking through doorways, entering an elevator, navigating small spaces, and making a turn. This suggests that there is a visuospatial component to freezing. Freezing may also occur when a person feels anxious or hurried. The harder one tries to break a freeze, the more difficult it becomes. A freeze can be managed with certain sensory cues. Each person will have a cue or combination of cues that works best for that person.

Assessment

Determine when freezing occurs in relationship to activity, the environment, time of day, and dosing of PD medications.

Item 14 on the UPDRS assesses freezing when walking and falling as related to freezing.

0 = Normal

1 = Rare freezing when walking, may have start hesitation

2 = Occasional freezing when walking

3 = Falls an average of once daily related to freezing

4 = Falls more than once daily related to freezing

Nonpharmacological Management

- Provide a referral to a physical therapist to assess freezing, provide gait training, and instruct the patient in how to use cueing and increase safety with ambulation.
- Share tips with the patient and family on how to break a freeze, as described in "Cueing Tips," in the next section.

Cuing Tips—General Strategies

- First, stop trying to continue the movement that elicits the freezing. Then, initiate a different movement. For example, if freezing occurs with walking, first stop walking and then try marching or reaching before resuming walking again.

Auditory

- Use a metronome or music, and walk to the beat. Bigger steps may help reduce freezing.
- Have a companion say, "Walk, march, and lift your leg."

Visual

- Look through, not directly at, doorways.
- Step over a marked line or spot on the floor.
- Use a device designed for gait freezing (such as a cane with a built-in apparatus to step over).
- Use a laser cane or a walker that emits a laser beam to step over.

Verbal

- Count one, two, three, four, five, out loud.
- March—left, right, left, right.

Pharmacological Management

- Sometimes, when a patient is undermedicated, increasing the dose of PD medications may alleviate freezing. If gait freezing occurs more during the "off" state, medication adjustments to relieve wearing off may help minimize this.

HALLUCINATIONS

Hallucinations are sensations that are perceived but are not real. They may affect one or more of the five primary senses: visual (seeing things or persons); auditory (hearing voices); tactile (feeling skin sensations); odorous (smelling nonexistent odors); and gustatory (appreciating an unusual taste).

In Parkinson's disease, hallucinations are almost always visual. They often consist of seeing small people, children, or animals, and are usually nonthreatening in nature. They are usually a side effect of the medication used to treat Parkinson symptoms or may occur if the person has an infection or ongoing toxic/metabolic encephalopathy. Older and cognitively impaired patients are more prone to this condition, but it can occur to any PD patient.

Hallucinations are more common late at night or early in the morning, when the person is falling asleep or upon awakening. Usually, the individual realizes that the hallucination is not real. However, some individuals believe they are real and are unable to distinguish the hallucinations from reality. When patients develop fixed beliefs about their hallucinations, they are considered to be delusional. When the delusions are accompanied by confusion, the person is in a state of psychosis. Individuals experiencing symptoms of psychosis need immediate medical attention. A visit to the hospital emergency room may be required because the individual may challenge the spouse/caregiver about these delusional beliefs, and may become suspicious, paranoid, and in rare situations, violent.

Typically, hallucinations occur later on in the illness and as a side effect of PD medications (in which all PD meds have been implicated). It is sometimes a fine balance between having too much medication and experiencing hallucinations versus having too little and experiencing worsening of PD symptoms. (See Figure 1.2.)

Hallucinations, if present early on in the course of the disease and not associated with anti-Parkinson medication, may suggest an atypical form of Parkinsonism called dementia with Lewy bodies (also known as Lewy body dementia).

Assessment

Patients and family members often do not report hallucinations without direct questioning. It is important to specifically ask them if

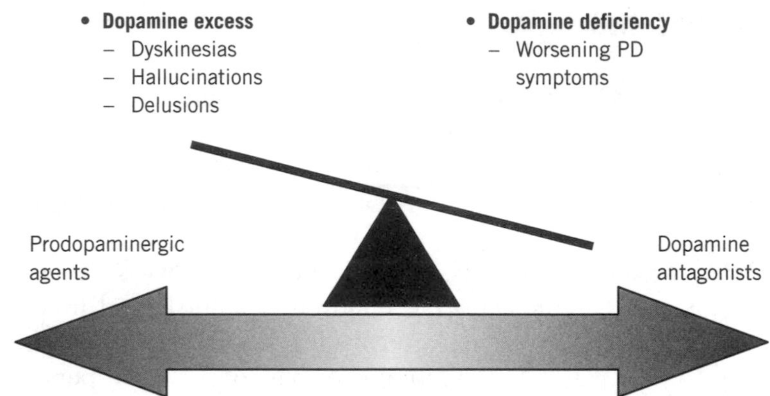

Figure 1.2 Complications of PD treatment.

hallucinations are present. Further inquiry should include a description of the hallucination, frequency, time of day, and relationship to medication. Ask if they are bothersome or frightening. Determine if any coexisting problems including sleep deprivation or infection are ongoing. These questions help determine the risk-to-benefit ratio of using certain Parkinson medications. They also help determine the need for an antipsychotic medication. For example, if hallucinations are mild and not bothersome to the patient, then perhaps only a slight adjustment in Parkinson medication is required or even no intervention at all.

Nonpharmacological Management

- Share information with the patient and family members to notify the physician about hallucinations, including onset after addition of a new medicine or change of dose, or if the severity of hallucinations increases.
- Provide reassurance to the patient and family that hallucinations are a side effect of Parkinson medication, not the fault of the person or family member.
- Role play is useful to teach family members how to respond during the actual hallucination. Gently reassuring the person that the hallucination is not real, that it is a side effect of the medication, and that the person is not losing his or her mind, is helpful.

Pharmacological Management

- A careful medication review is needed with the patient's physician, as the hallucinations may lessen or go away if it can be determined if a potentially responsible medication can be decreased or discontinued. Typically, the neurologist may need to simplify a patient's PD regimen when a patient is hallucinating and "peel off" anti-PD meds one at a time until the hallucinations disappear or further simplification results in worsening of motor symptoms. (See Figure 1.3.)
- Atypical antipsychotics are used to treat moderate to severe hallucinations. Two atypical antipsychotics may be useful: quetiapine (Seroquel®) and clozapine (Clozaril®). Nearly all other antipsychotics, including the ones labeled as "atypical" such as olanzapine (Zyprexa®), risperidone (Risperdal®), aripiprazole (Abilify®), and so forth, may control hallucinations but can worsen Parkinson's disease symptoms significantly and should be avoided.
- The dose of the atypical antipsychotic is often low initially and is slowly increased to treat symptoms and to lessen the chance of side effects such as sleepiness, light-headedness, and weight gain. To assess the presence of orthostatic hypotension, blood pressure and pulse are measured in the supine position and after standing for one minute. These measurements should be obtained at the start of the medication and at intervals throughout treatment.

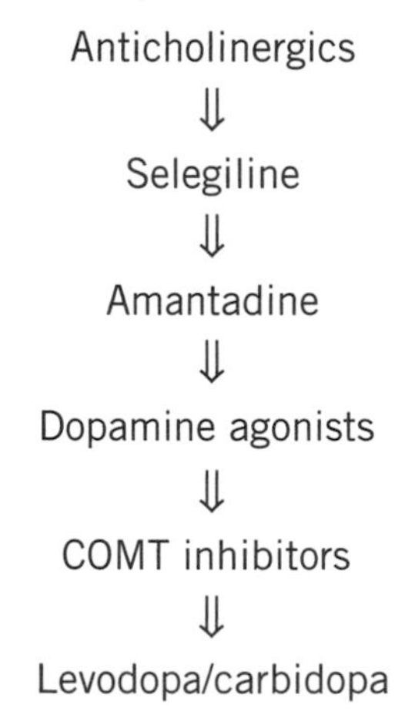

Figure 1.3 Priority of modification.
From "The Role of Atypical Antipsychotics in the Treatment of Movement Disorders," by H. H. Fernandez & J. H. Friedman, 1999. *CNS Drugs, 11*(6), 467–483.

- Clozapine (Clozaril®) has the potential to cause a severe drop in the white blood cell (WBC) count in 1%–2% of individuals. The Food and Drug Administration requires weekly blood counts for six months. These are then decreased to every other week for six months and monthly thereafter.

LEG SWELLING

Swelling of the legs can occur due to a variety of reasons including poor drainage from veins or lymphatic vessels, excessive fluid accumulation from heart failure, venous thrombosis, kidney problems, and certain medications. In Parkinson's disease, leg swelling is reported often by patients and may be due to decreased mobility, or most often is a side effect of PD medications. The medications that increase the likelihood of leg swelling include amantadine and dopamine agonists such as pramipexole (Mirapex®), ropinirole (Requip®), and apomorphine (Apokyn®). In addition, fludrocortisone (Florinef®) used to treat orthostatic hypotension can cause leg swelling.

Assessment

Medical history and physical examination should follow any report of leg swelling. Venous thrombosis (thrombophlebitis, blood clot) requires immediate attention. Leg swelling associated with thrombosis is usually accompanied by pain, especially calf tenderness, and typically affects only one leg. A Doppler ultrasound may be ordered by the physician to rule this out.

A cardiac and kidney workup may be ordered to rule out other causes of leg swelling.

Nonpharmacological Management

Once it has been determined that leg swelling is related to Parkinson symptoms or PD medications, patient and family education should be done and include instructions to:

- Elevate legs during sitting periods.
- Avoid prolonged sitting: periodically get up and walk around. This is particularly important when traveling long distances, especially by plane.

- Wear compressive hose. Compressive hose, such as Jobst® stockings, will constrict leg veins and limit swelling. Hose must fit properly to be effective. They should be put on in the morning when swelling is at a minimum.
- Decrease salt in the diet.
- Attend a lymphedema clinic. Some hospitals specialize in treating moderate to severe leg swelling. This often includes performance of a variety of tests accompanied by wrapping techniques, massage, and hygiene of the affected limb(s), as well as therapeutic and remedial exercises.

Pharmacological Management

- Review medication list and revise as appropriate. Discuss risk-benefit ratio with the patient. Sometimes changing the type of dopamine agonist or eliminating amantadine is useful.
- Physicians often prescribe a diuretic to treat swelling. These medications may lower potassium levels, creating a need for potassium supplementation or consumption of a daily banana (which contains potassium). Other disadvantages of diuretics are that they cause increased urination, which can disrupt sleep. Furthermore, they can lower blood pressure, which can aggravate light-headedness and precipitate fainting if the individual already has low blood pressures such as may occur with orthostatic hypotension.

MICROGRAPHIA

Fine motor coordination is affected by loss of hand dexterity, increased muscle tone, and tremor. Micrographia is the very small handwriting observed in Parkinson's disease. People typically report that when writing, the words progressively get smaller and smaller. Handwriting may be illegible.

Assessment

Rate handwriting in a person's "on" state and "off" using item 8 of the UPDRS:

0 = normal

1 = slightly slow or small

2 = moderately slow or small; all words are legible

3 = severely affected; not all words are legible

4 = the majority of words are not legible

Nonpharmacological Management

- Provide a referral to an occupational therapist to address upper-body movement and fine motor coordination.

Advise Patients to

- Use adaptive devices including built-up pen grips
- Perform writing tasks when mobility is optimal
- Explore other methods of recording information including use of computer word processing programs
- Use preprinted name and address labels when unable to write

Pharmacological Management

- Sometimes, micrographia is worsened when the patient is undermedicated or in the wearing-off state. Adjustment of PD medications may improve this condition.

MOTOR FLUCTUATIONS

As Parkinson's disease progresses, responses to levodopa or dopamine agonists become less consistent and motor fluctuations develop. This typically occurs 4–7 years after the initiation of levodopa. Motor fluctuations include wearing off, "on-off," dyskinesia, and dystonia. The cause of motor fluctuations is not completely understood, but it is hypothesized that they are related to the intermittent delivery of levodopa. Efforts are under way to develop products that will provide continuous delivery of levodopa or continuous dopaminergic stimulation.

Wearing-Off Effect

Wearing off is a shortened duration of the effectiveness of each dose. Patients notice that a medication dose does not last as long as it once did.

For example, a patient took a carbidopa/levodopa dose at 7:00 A.M. and noted benefit (relief of rigidity, tremor, and slowness) by 8:00 A.M. Previously he or she was symptom free until 11:00 A.M. when he or she took the next dose. However, because of wearing off, the patient has noticed at 10:00 A.M. the return of stiffness, difficulty with fine motor movement, and tremor.

"On-Off" Effect

"On-off" effect is a rapid change between the "on" state (a period of symptom relief and good mobility) and the "off" state (a return of Parkinson symptoms with decreased mobility). For example, a person takes a 4:00 P.M. dose of carbidopa/levodopa and it begins to work effectively at 4:30 P.M. This person expected two hours of symptom relief but at 4:45 P.M. has a sudden unpredictable "off" period.

Dyskinesia

Dyskinesia is the involuntary writhing choreiform movement that may be observed in the face, limbs, neck, or trunk. It can be very subtle or mild, only recognized by an experienced observer, or moderate to severe, causing significant disability. Dyskinesia most often occurs at the peak dose when medication is most effective, but may occur at other times in the dosing schedule.

Dystonia

Dystonia is a sustained muscle contraction that is often described as a cramp. It can occur as part of the disease process of PD or as a complication of medication. Individuals commonly report dystonia of the foot (toe curling) or leg, which is usually worse in the morning before the first dose of medication.

Assessment

- Perform a complete medical history and physical examination.
- Utilize patient diaries to keep track of motor fluctuations at home. Diaries should include time of medication dose and an hourly report of symptoms. The diary is useful in monitoring motor states. It is useful because it allows the patient to report if dyskinesia is

troublesome (interferes with function or causes meaningful discomfort) or nontroublesome (does not interfere with function or cause meaningful discomfort).

- The UPDRS includes the following items related to motor fluctuations and complications of therapy:

Dyskinesia

0= None

1 = 1%–25% of day

2 = 26%–50% of day

3 = 51%–75% of day

4 = 76%–100% of day

Disability: How Disabling Is Dyskinesia?

0 = Not disabling

1 = Mildly disabling

2 = Moderately disabling

3 = Severely disabling

4 = Completely disabling

Painful Dyskinesia: How Painful Is the Dyskinesia?

0 = Not painful

1 = Slightly

2 = Moderately

3 = Severely

4 = Markedly

Presence of Early Morning Dystonia

Are any "off" periods predictable as to timing after a dose of medication? (0 = No, 1= Yes)

Are any "off" periods unpredictable as to timing after a dose of medication? (0 = No, 1= Yes)

Do any "off" periods come on suddenly? (0 = No, 1= Yes)

What proportion of the waking day is the subject "off" on average?

0 = None

1 = 1%–25% of day

2 = 26%–50% of day

3 = 51%–75% of day

4 = 76%–100% of day

Pharmacological Management

- Provide the patient with a clearly written schedule of medications. Instruct the patient and family to administer medications on time and as scheduled. Prefilled pill boxes and medication timers will improve compliance.
- Provide an individualized medication schedule. Medication adjustments to treat motor fluctuations are individualized and depend on many factors including history of medication response, side-effect profile, and comorbidities.
- Adjust the timing of carbidopa/levodopa (Sinemet®) doses; move them closer together as needed.
- Add the dopamine agonists pramipexole (Mirapex®) or ropinirole (Requip®) to the medication regimen. Apomorphine (Apokyn®) is very useful for sudden "on-off" effect.
- Add COMT inhibitors (entacapone, Comtan®) (Stalevo®) to increase "on" time.
- Add monoamine oxidase B (MAO-B) inhibitors selegiline (Eldepryl®) or rasagiline (Azilect®) to increase "on" time.
- Reduce dose of anti-PD medications to decrease dyskinesia.
- Amantadine (Symmetrel®) provides partial reduction of dyskinesias; dosing often begins with 100 mg BID, then can be increased to 100 mg TID as needed.
- Consider referral of the patient to participate in a clinical research trial designed to improve motor fluctuations.

- Provide the patient and family with information on deep brain stimulation (DBS) surgery. Refer as appropriate. (See Table 1.1.)

Nonpharmacological Management

- Assist patient with care during "off" periods.
- Provide information to the patient and family on skilled and non-skilled home care services. Complete a referral as appropriate.

Table 1.1

TREATMENT OF MOTOR FLUCTUATIONS

MOTOR FLUCTUATION	USUAL TREATMENT OPTIONS	OTHER TREATMENT CONSIDERATIONS
Wearing "off"	Increase frequency and/or dose of levodopa administration Add rasagiline Add orally disintegrating selegiline Add dopamine agonist Controlled release levodopa Add COMT inhibitor Add MAO inhibitor Add amantadine	Dietary manipulation
"On-off" fluctuations	Add apomorphine Consider deep brain stimulation surgery	Duodenal levodopa pump (not yet approved in the United States)
Dose failures	Consider apomorphine	Improve gastric empyting
Freezing	Levodopa Physical therapy Visual cues	Use MAO-B inhibitors Try dopamine agonists
"Off" period Dystonia	Levodopa	Consider clozapine
Peak-dose dyskinesia	Decrease dosage of levodopa Add dopamine agonist while decreasing levodopa Amantadine Consider deep brain stimulation surgery	Consider clozapine

- Provide information and instruction to the patient and family on relaxation therapy. This may be particularly useful during "off" periods
- Evaluate the patient's ability to safely ambulate, drive, and perform activities of daily living with motor fluctuations. Counsel the patient/family as appropriate.

NUMBNESS AND TINGLING

Numbness and tingling, called *paresthesias,* are abnormal sensations that can occur in the body, and are often felt in the hands, feet, arms, or legs. Individuals with Parkinson's disease often experience this symptom.

There are many possible causes:

- Parkinson's disease may be accompanied by altered sensations on the side of the body where the Parkinson symptoms initially begin.
- Nerve compression from remaining in the same position for prolonged periods of time, such as sitting in a car, may cause paresthesias. Nerve compression can also occur from overuse such as doing repetitive wrist movements that can cause carpal tunnel syndrome. In this condition there may be numbness/tingling in the hand and fingers that often awakens the person at night.
- With a neck or back injury there may be pain and altered sensation along the course of the nerve to an arm, hand, foot, or leg. For example, with a low-back injury and a herniated disk, sciatica may occur, which manifests as a sensation of numbness or tingling down the back of the leg along with back pain or leg pain.
- Individuals who have significant arthritis of the back called spinal stenosis can develop numbness and leg pain that occur with walking (called neurogenic claudication). The patient with this condition usually can walk longer distances pushing a shopping cart (when stooped over) before the symptoms appear.
- Another condition that can occur with walking is called vascular or vasogenic claudication. This disorder is due to atherosclerotic disease from plaque buildup in the arteries to the legs. With walking there is insufficient blood supply and the person experiences pain, numbness, and tingling while walking that soon resolves after stopping to rest.

- Nerve pathology called neuropathy can be caused by many diseases such as diabetes, thyroid conditions, vitamin B-12 deficiencies, radiation injury, kidney failure, or other disorders.
- Brain disorders such as stroke, multiple sclerosis, and even seizures and migraine can be accompanied by altered sensations in the body.
- Altered electrolytes can alter sensation as well.

Assessment

Numerous tests can be performed; however, the history usually provides clues as to where to look for the problem, starting with the brain, spinal cord, nerve roots, and peripheral nerves.

Diagnostic tests that may be performed include:

- Blood tests such as CBC, electrolytes, thyroid function tests, and vitamin B-12 levels
- Imaging studies: CT or MRI of the head or spine
- Electromyogram (EMG) to evaluate peripheral nerve and muscle function
- Plain film X-rays
- Lumbar puncture (spinal tap) to look for infection, inflammation, and so forth

Management

Treatment is dependent on the underlying cause. Individuals with Parkinson's should be reminded to change position frequently to avoid nerve compression. Sometimes, when the paresthesias become really bothersome, medications are given to alleviate the discomfort. (See Table 1.2.)

ORTHOSTATIC HYPOTENSION (LOW BLOOD PRESSURE)

Orthostatic hypotension (OH) is a substantial drop in blood pressure upon standing as compared to seated or lying pressures. Classically OH is present when there is a drop greater than 30 mm Hg systolic or 15 mg diastolic from lying to standing position. Crucial to OH is whether there are symptoms that accompany the drop and these most often consist of light-headedness, or dizziness, and fainting. Other symptoms include

Table 1.2

PHARMACOLOGIC THERAPY FOR NEUROPATHIC PAIN

THERAPY	STARTING DOSES	MAINTENANCE DOSES
Bupropion	150 mg a day	After one week, increase to 150 mg BID
Carbamazepine	200 mg BID	Increase by 200-mg increments to 200–400 mg 3–4 times a day; follow drug level on doses greater than 600 mg a day
Duloxetine	30 mg a day	Increase by 30–60-mg increments up to 120 mg a day
Gabapentin	300 mg TID	Increase by 300–400-mg increments to 2,400–6,000 mg daily divided in 3–4 doses
Lamotrigine	25 mg QD or BID	Increase by 25-mg increments weekly to 100–200 mg BID
Levetiracetam	250 mg at bedtime	Increase by 250–500-mg increments to 1,500 mg BID
Mexiletine	200 mg once a day	Increase by 200-mg increments to a maximum of 200 mg TID
Oxcarbazepine	150–300 mg BID	Increase by 300-mg increments to 600–1,200 mg BID
Pregabalin	50 mg TID	Increase to 300 mg per day
Phenytoin	200 mg at bedtime	Increase by 100-mg increments to 300–400 mg daily divided in 1–2 doses, following drug levels
Tiagabine	4 mg a day	Increase to 4–12 mg BID
Tramadol	50 mg BID or TID	Increase by 50-mg increments to a maximum of 100 mg QID
Tricyclic anti-depressants	10–25 mg at bedtime	Increase by 10–25-mg increments to 100–150 mg at bedtime
Topiramate	25–50 mg at bedtime	Increase by 50-mg increments weekly to 200 mg BID
Venlafaxine XR	37.5–75 mg QD	Increase by 75-mg increments to 150–225 mg a day
Zonisamide	100 mg at bedtime	Increase by 100-mg increments to 400–600 mg at bedtime

fatigue and confusion. In PD, blood pressure changes are most often due to autonomic nervous system impairment and/or the use of anti-Parkinson medications. Some individuals who have orthostatic hypotension may also experience intermittent high blood pressure, usually while in the supine position, and at night.

Individuals with significant orthostatic hypotension, particularly if it occurs early in the disease, should be evaluated for multiple system atrophy (MSA), a condition which also has many features of idiopathic Parkinson's disease. However, a milder form of OH can be seen in some patients with PD. More commonly, OH in PD is due to medication side effects. Most medications have been implicated, but in particular, dopamine agonists, levodopa, amantadine, and anticholinergic medications.

Blood pressure monitoring is important to ensure that orthostatic hypotension is being treated adequately but not so overtreated that the blood pressure goes too high. Patients should purchase a home blood-pressure monitor. The patient and family member(s) should be taught how and when to use it, and to check both the lying and standing values. A common mistake is to record only a seated pressure, which obviously misses the crucial issue of a blood pressure drop that occurs when the person rises to a standing position.

Blood pressure is lowest in the morning and drops in blood pressure are typically the greatest at this time, so it is a good time to do the readings. A pulse measurement should also be recorded. Consider checking the blood pressure and pulse at other times of the day such as after breakfast, in the afternoon after lunch, and at bedtime. This consistent checking may give a sense of the degree of variability in blood pressure that occurs throughout the day. In addition to just recording numbers it is important also to record how the person feels when blood pressure is measured. Not everyone who has a large drop in blood pressure feels dizzy or has other symptoms from OH, and therefore not everyone needs to be treated. Nonetheless, taken together, if the person has significant OH and is symptomatic, he or she may need to be treated. Keep in mind that patients with cognitive impairment may not be able to report their OH symptoms.

Assessment

- Routinely assess all PD patients for orthostatic hypotension.
- Monitor BP and heart rate in supine, sitting, and standing positions. Have patient supine for 5 minutes; then take BP and pulse.

Have patient sit for 1 minute; record BP and pulse. Have patient stand for 2 minutes and then record BP and pulse.

- Perform medical history and physical exam to rule out other causes of orthostatic hypotension.
- Provide careful assessment of medications used for Parkinson's disease and coexisting health problems. Note what medications may decrease or increase BP, and then consult with the primary health care provider.
- Refer the patient to an autonomic specialist to provide a comprehensive evaluation of blood pressure, sweating, bladder function, and response to medication. Many autonomic laboratories or centers employ both a cardiologist and a neurologist. For moderate to severe orthostatic hypotension, testing may include the following:
  - Tilt-table testing is used to evaluate for changes in blood pressure and heart rate in different positions.
  - Electrocardiogram (ECG), cardiac rhythm monitoring with a Holter monitor, and cardiac electrophysiological studies may mean it would be wise to look for abnormal heart rhythm as a cause for fainting spells.
  - Blood studies (such as a complete blood count or CBC) are done to assess for anemia.
  - Endocrinological tests, such as cortisol, assess the possibility of adrenal dysfunction.

Nonpharmacological Management

Instruct patient/family member to:

- Purchase and correctly use a home blood-pressure monitor.
- Properly rise from a seated position. The patient should sit on the edge of the bed or a chair for a few minutes, and then stand up slowly, holding onto something stable for a few seconds before attempting to walk.
- Sleep with the head of the bed elevated about 6–8 inches.
- Use compression/support hose (Jobst®) stockings during the day.
- Elevate legs periodically during the day.
- Increase fluids (at least 8 glasses of water per day).
- Increase salt and caffeine in the diet.

- Eat five small meals a day because blood pressure is lowered after a large meal.
- Avoid hot showers or excessive heat.

Pharmacological Management

- Adjust all medications to decrease orthostatic hypotension. Dopamine agonists should be slowly titrated down, if possible.
- Occasionally salt tablets or other medications including fludrocortisone and proamatine are prescribed. It is important that fludrocortisone be given in the morning, and proamitine not be given later than 6 P.M., to avoid supine hypertension when patients go to bed to retire for the night.
- Fludrocortisone (Florinef®): Fludrocortisone increases circulation volume, which helps elevate blood pressure. As the dose is increased there may be excessive fluid retention that can cause swelling in the feet/legs as well as heart failure resulting in shortness of breath. Electrolyte monitoring is needed, as a drop in potassium can occur that may require supplemental potassium pills or the need for a daily banana (which contains potassium).
- Midodrine (ProAmatine®): midodrine is an alpha-1 adrenergic agonist that causes increased blood pressure through vasoconstriction. As mentioned, midodrine should not be taken too late in the day so as not to cause hypertension in the evening. Often midodrine is taken with fludrocortisone.
- Other medications that may help orthostatic hypotension include:
  - Methylphenidate (Ritalin®)
  - Octreotide (Sandostatin®)
  - Propranolol (Inderal®), or other beta-blockers
  - Pyridostigmine (Mestinon®)
  - Theophylline (Theo-Dur®)
  - Venlafaxine (Effexor®)
  - Fluoxetine (Prozac®)
  - Indomethacin (Indocin®)

PAIN IN PARKINSON'S DISEASE

Individuals with Parkinson's disease do experience pain. It may be from a symptom directly related to PD such as a painful dystonic cramp. It may be related to a condition caused by a symptom of PD, such as a painful frozen shoulder from rigidity and decreased mobility, or an injury resulting from a fall caused by gait abnormalities or postural instability. Finally, it may be a health problem unrelated to PD but often made worse by PD. An example of this is pain from a radiculopathy that may increase with rigidity or with the involuntary movements of dyskinesia.

This section will describe some of the common pain syndromes that occur in PD.

Spinal Stenosis

Spinal stenosis is a narrowing of the spinal canal that can cause compression of the spinal cord and/or nerve roots. Typically it occurs in the lower back (lumbar region) or in the neck (cervical spine). Degenerative arthritis of the spine is the most common cause for this condition. A person with lumbar spinal stenosis may have back pain and notice that he or she can walk longer distances by taking frequent breaks, or by walking bent over (for example when pushing a shopping cart), because this posture mechanically lessens stenosis. Therefore a stooped posture may be seen with aging due to spinal stenosis or Parkinson's disease; they commonly coexist.

Radiculopathy (Nerve Root Problem)

Impingement or compression of a nerve root is called a *radiculopathy*. Typically radiculopathy is painful (often described as shooting pains from the low back down the leg or from the neck down the arms or fingers) and may be accompanied by weakness or numbness. One common radiculopathy involving the low back is called *sciatica,* wherein the person usually has radiating pain down one leg below the knee. The radiating pain is often worsened by coughing, sneezing, and bearing down, as well as prolonged standing or sitting.

Neuropathy

Symptoms of peripheral neuropathy include numbness, tingling, and painful paresthesias in the hands and/or feet in a "glove and stocking" fashion. Neuropathic pain occurs because nerve fibers themselves are damaged or dysfunctional. These damaged nerve fibers send signals to pain centers. Damage or dysfunction in the spinal cord or, rarely, in the brain can also cause neuropathic pain. Some common conditions with neuropathic pain include diabetes, shingles, or multiple sclerosis.

Neuropathic pain can be very disabling because it may not respond to standard analgesic medications. Sometimes narcotics are used as well as medications that are used to treat epilepsy, that is, anticonvulsant compounds, such as gabapentin, carbamazepine, pregabalin, and so on.

Painful Dystonia

Dystonia are prolonged or sustained involuntary muscle contractions that result in abnormal posturing of the involved body part. In Parkinson's they can occur in any limb, the face, neck, and trunk. They can be part of the disease process or be caused by the medication used to treat PD. Some individuals experience early morning dystonia. These sharp cramps occur most often in the legs and feet. They are described as a very painful charley horse that does not immediately resolve and can last up to several hours. Individuals with dystonia report pain ranging from minimal pain to severe pain. Dystonia occurs more often in people with young-onset Parkinson's disease.

Assessment

Pain assessment should occur at every patient visit.

A complete medical history of pain should include:

- Time of onset
- Location
- Description
- Intensity
- Specific triggers
- What relieves pain
- Relationship to Parkinson symptoms
- Relationship to PD medications

Physical examination may demonstrate weakness, altered sensation, and/or changes in reflexes. Investigations may include:

- X-ray of the spine to look for a fracture, narrowing of the spinal canal as seen with spinal stenosis, and an assortment of other degenerative changes.
- Spinal MRI or CT to look for disease of the spine, disks, spinal cord, and nerve roots.

- Electromyography (EMG) examination, which may show signs of a nerve-root injury or a neuropathy and at times can help sort out if there are active or chronic changes.
- Certain blood tests performed to identify the underlying cause of a peripheral neuropathy.

Treatment will depend on numerous factors including type of pain, location, duration, relationship to Parkinson symptoms, and treatment.

Nonpharmacological Management

- Instruct patient to use a heating pad or ice packs.
- Instruct the patient and family caregiver on proper body mechanics. For lower back pain, bend at the knees and not at the waist. Keep the weight near the body when carrying objects. For neck pain, work at eye level.
- Provide a referral to physical therapy such as ultrasound therapy, cervical traction, and massage therapy. Exercises may be appropriate for some people to improve muscle strength.
- Provide a referral to an occupational therapist to evaluate and treat repetitive movement injuries, assess need for assistive devices, and vocational and occupational counseling.
- Refer patient to a psychologist to try cognitive-behavioral therapy or mindfulness-based therapy. These are treatments designed to help people in pain reduce the distress associated with pain.
- Consider nerve stimulation. Various devices use electric impulses to help block or mask the feeling of pain. With transcutaneous electrical nerve stimulation (TENS), a portable, battery-powered unit delivers an electric impulse through electrodes placed on the affected area. Spinal cord and peripheral nerve stimulators are implanted beneath the skin with electrodes placed near the spinal cord. A handheld unit is adjustable to allow for control of the level of stimulation.
- Provide referral to a pain specialist when pain is not responding to conventional therapies.
- Refer the patient for surgical evaluation. Most cases of radiculopathy respond to pharmacologic treatment and resolve within 30 to 90 days. However, excruciating pain or persistent pain may require surgical intervention if impingement of a specific root is identified. Similarly, spinal stenosis may require surgical correction.

Pharmacological Management

- Parkinson medications should be adjusted to treat pain related to PD symptoms or complications of therapy (such as painful wearing off).
- Use over-the-counter analgesics (e.g., acetaminophen, ibuprofen) to control pain.
- Use prescription analgesics to control moderate to severe pain. These may include codeine, hydrocodone, fentanyl patch, and so forth. PD patients are at increased risk of constipation and confusion with these medications.
- Botulinum toxin injections can be useful in treating some pain syndromes associated with dystonia.
- Steroid injections can be used to reduce inflammation around a nerve.
- Phenytoin, carbamazepine, or tricyclic antidepressants such as amitriptyline may also reduce nerve pain.
- Some physicians inject medication directly into the affected area as a supplement to medication therapy. Such injections are usually a combination of a numbing agent (local anesthetic), which provides immediate relief, and a corticosteroid, which reduces inflammation.
- An implantable medication pump supplies pain medication directly into the spinal fluid. To replenish the pump, drugs are injected through the skin into a small port at the center of the pump.

POSTURAL INSTABILITY

Postural instability, the inability to maintain balance, is one of the cardinal features of Parkinson's disease. It usually does not appear until later in the disease. Individuals with postural instability are at risk for falls that may lead to bruising, fractures, or head injury.

Falls may occur early in the disease due to a misstep or shuffling gait. Individuals with orthostatic hypotension, moderate to severe dyskinesia, or who have neurocognitive difficulties including increased impulsivity or memory problems are also at risk of falling. These issues have a significant impact on the mobility and quality of life of patients as well as increasing morbidity.

Assessment

- A medical history and a physical exam should be done to assess balance, and also frequency and triggers of falls.
- Postural instability is examined by using the pull test. The examiner stands behind the patient and pulls back sharply on the patient's shoulders; the patient's eyes should be open and feet slightly apart. Patients are asked to correct themselves and usually will need to take one or two steps to do so. The UPDRS includes an item on postural stability:

  0 = Normal

  1 = Retropulsion, but recovers unaided

  2 = Absence of postural response; would fall if not caught by examiner

  3 = Very unstable; tends to lose balance spontaneously

  4 = Unable to stand without assistance

Nonpharmacological Management

- Provide referral to a physical therapist for evaluation and treatment including fall prevention, balance training, exercise, and recommendations for safety and the proper use of assistive devices.
- Provide patient/family information on home safety including:
  - Removing throw rugs
  - Adding handrails
  - Improving lighting
  - Removing clutter to clear a pathway

Pharmacological Management

- Postural instability does not usually respond to medication adjustment. However, medications can be optimized to decrease dyskinesia, confusion, or orthostatic hypotension.

PSYCHOSIS

Psychoses can occur in individuals with advanced Parkinson's disease and also in those with chronic exposure to anti-Parkinson medications.

Psychotic symptoms may also be observed early in the disease process of individuals diagnosed with diffuse Lewy body dementia, an atypical form of parkinsonism. In PD, visual hallucinations are the most common manifestation, occurring in approximately 30%–50% of individuals. Patients describe these hallucinations as well formed, such as seeing small children or animals that appear to move. Although PD patients with hallucinations typically have intact reality testing (*benign hallucinosis*), at least 5% of patients experience delusions and hallucinations unaccompanied by insight. These individuals often exhibit paranoia, agitation, and increased confusion. This latter population with psychosis contributes to higher caregiver strain, increased rates of nursing home placement, and a dramatically dimmer prognosis in extended care facilities.

Assessment

Patients and family members often do not report hallucinations or other behavioral problems associated with psychosis without direct questioning, or until the episodes cannot be managed at home. It is important to ask them specifically if hallucinations are present. Further inquiries should include descriptions of the hallucination, frequency, time of day, and relationship to medications. It should be asked if the hallucinations are bothersome or frightening. Investigate to see if there is an associated paranoia. Spouses are often accused of infidelity and have great difficulty coping with this accusation. Identify any coexisting problems, including sleep deprivation or infection, that may be taking place. This identification helps determine the risk-to-benefit ratio of using certain Parkinson medications as well as the need for antipsychotic medications. Safety evaluation and plans need to be discussed with family members or health care professionals if individuals are residing in health care settings.

Pharmacological Management

- A careful medication review is needed, as hallucinations may lessen or resolve if an offending medication can be decreased or stopped.
- Atypical antipsychotics are used to treat moderate to severe hallucinations. Two atypical antipsychotics may be useful and include quetiapine (Seroquel®) and clozapine (Clozaril®). Nearly all other antipsychotics may control hallucinations but can worsen Parkinson's disease symptoms significantly and should be avoided.

ften started initially as a symptoms and to lessen iness, light-headedness, of orthostatic hypoten- measured in the supine of the medication, then

to cause a severe drop in 6–2% of individuals. The weekly blood counts for eased to every other week See Table 1.3.)

Table 1.3

YCHOSIS

			CE OF Y	TENDENCY TO WORSEN PARKINSONISM
Clozapine	Antipsychotic	24.7–36	Proven	Minimal
Risperidone	Antipsychotic	0.7–1.9	Best avoided	Significant
Olanzapine	Antipsychotic	4.1–6.5	Best avoided	Moderate
Quetiapine	Antipsychotic	54–200	Probably helpful	Mild
Aripiprazole	Antipsychotic	1–12	Unproven	Variable
Ziprasidone	Antipsychotic	N/A	Unproven	Moderate
Tacrine	Cholinesterase inhibitor	40–60	Unproven	Variable
Donepezil	Cholinesterase inhibitor	5–10	Possibly helpful	Minimal
Galantamine	Cholinesterase inhibitor	4–8	Possibly helpful	Unclear
Rivastigmine	Cholinesterase inhibitor	1.5–8.9	Possibly helpful	Minimal
Ondansetron	Antiemetic	12–24	Unproven	Minimal

Nonpharmacological Management

- Implement safety measures to prevent injury. Confused patients may become agitated and/or combative. Psychosis has caused individuals to fall out of bed, escape from their immediate surroundings, leave their homes, and even drive. Occasionally, restraints, alarm mats, or other measures may be necessary to ensure safety. A restraint plan must be ordered by a physician, signed by a health care proxy, and closely monitored by a health care provider. Some individuals will require a sitter to provide constant supervision.
- Provide emotional support to the patient and family members during this difficult time. Referral to a mental health care professional is useful for the family caregiver if the patient's confusion is chronic. Family caregivers may also benefit from support groups that include members coping with similar experiences.

SEBORRHEIC DERMATITIS

Seborrheic dermatitis is a skin condition common in individuals with Parkinson's disease. It can be present on all skin areas and is most recognized as oily, chafed, reddened skin over the eyebrows, forehead, and scalp. For men, skin changes may also develop over the beard area. The scaly, inflamed skin can be itchy or painful to touch. It can also involve temporary hair loss if the dermatitis is located on the scalp.

The exact cause of seborrheic dermatitis is unknown. It is thought to be common in people with Parkinson's disease due to an increased secretion of sebum by hair follicles. The skin abnormalities can partly improve with the use of carbidopa/levodopa, but typically other remedies are required.

Assessment

All individuals with Parkinson's disease should have an annual skin evaluation by a dermatologist to evaluate and treat seborrhea and most importantly to identify precancerous or cancerous skin lesions (basal cell carcinoma, squamous cell carcinoma, or melanoma).

Evaluate individual's ability to perform self-skin care. Practicing good hygiene may be impaired due to decreased mobility.

Nonpharmacological Management

Counsel patient and family education to:

- Use over-the-counter dandruff shampoos containing selenium sulfide (Selsun Blue®, Head & Shoulders®), salicylic acid (X-Seb®, Scalpicin Ionil®, Plus®, P&S®), or coal tar (Ionil T®, DHS Tar®, Neutrogena T/Gel®, Polytar®) to help control itching and flaking. When using a dandruff shampoo, rub the shampoo into the hair thoroughly and let it stay on hair and scalp for at least 3 minutes before rinsing.
- Emphasize the importance of keeping the skin clean and dry at all times.

Pharmacological Management

- Hydrocortisone cream 1% is available over the counter and may be massaged into the scalp or applied to scaly skin patches once or twice daily. This should be used for a short term only under the guidance of a health care provider.
- A prescription cream or shampoo, 2% ketoconazole, can also help in some cases.
- Prescription drug treatment includes the use of selenium (Selsun®), pimecrolimus (Elidel®), tacrolimus (Protopic®), and topical cortisone-like drugs, such as betamethasone (Diprosone lotion®) and fluocinonide (Lidex®, Capex® solution). Protopic® and Elidel® should only be used for a short term as safe chronic use has not been established.

SELF-CARE DEFICIT

Changes in fine- and gross-motor skills, cognition, and mood impact one's ability to perform activities of daily living (ADLs). Rigidity, slowness of movement, tremor, postural instability, fatigue, and depression are a few of the PD symptoms that interfere with a person's functional capabilities. For example, decreased trunk mobility and abnormal motor initiation will make it difficult when turning and when getting in and out of bed.

PD medications and other treatments significantly improve functional ability. However, over time, a worsening of symptoms as well as unpredictable motor fluctuations will challenge one's ability to manage self-care. Family and health care providers require a special understanding that many people with PD have fluctuations in their mobility throughout the day. Typically these fluctuations follow a dosing cycle. The person with PD may be independent at the peak effect of a medication dose, but 2 hours later may require complete assistance.

Humans have an innate desire to care for themselves. In order to accomplish this, individuals with Parkinson's must have support from qualified and insightful health care professionals. With this guidance, patients will be able to deal effectively with those challenges along the self-care continuum from meeting their own physical needs through to managing psychosocial concerns.

Assessment

- A complete history and evaluation of the person's ability to complete activities of daily living should be done. An occupational therapist is specially trained in the evaluation of ADLs.
- Any evaluation should include the time of day, when PD medications were taken, and the person's dose response and motor state ("on" or "off"). An individual will have more difficulty performing ADLs in the "off" state.
- Areas of ADL function to be assessed include dressing, hygiene, toileting, meal preparation, feeding, bed and transfer mobility, handwriting and keyboarding, homemaking, manipulation of money, and participation in work and leisure activities.

Nonpharmacological Management

- Provide referral to an occupational therapist for evaluation and treatment of functional impairment of ADLs.
- Use assistive devices to increase autonomy in ADL performance. Some examples include using built-up pen grips and eating utensils, Velcro on clothing and purse, and a mobility transfer handle for turning in bed.
- Encourage the patient to perform more difficult tasks when movement is easier and medications are working well.
- Always encourage independence and autonomy but assist patients in realizing limitations and in seeking assistance when necessary.
- Assess family for caregiver strain.

- Provide referral to home care agencies to provide services to assist patient/family with personal care and homemaking.
- Offer emotional support and counseling to patients dealing with a loss of independence.

Pharmacological Management

- Optimize PD medications to decrease disabling symptoms.
- Schedule medications in relationship to ADLs. For example, taking PD medications 30–60 minutes before eating may improve the mobility required to feed independently.

Patient/Family Resources

www.buyhandybar.com—An assistive device to get in and out of the car easily.

www.caregiverproducts.com—Provides in-home care aids for people with Parkinson's disease.

Cianci, H., Cloete, L., Gardner, J., Trail, M., & Wichman, R. (2006). *Activities of daily living: Practical pointers for Parkinson disease* (3rd ed.). Miami, FL: National Parkinson Foundation. Suggestions for maintaining independence in, and use of adaptive aides for, bathing, dressing, sleeping, eating, toileting, and mobility. Includes helpful tips for caregivers. Publication of the National Parkinson Foundation, www.parkinson.org

Clapcich, J., Goldberg, N., & Walsh, E. (2008). *Be independent: Equipment and suggestions for daily living activities.* New York: American Parkinson Disease Association. www.apdaparkinson.org

SEXUAL DYSFUNCTION

Sexual dysfunction may involve a reduction in sex drive with difficulty becoming aroused, difficulty achieving and sustaining an erection, inability to achieve orgasm, or pain with sexual activity or intercourse. Individuals may also experience dysfunction due to immobility. There are many causes, some attributed to Parkinson's, others related to coexisting conditions.

Rarely, PD patients will actually experience increase in libido and sometimes increase in sexual activity more than their norm, a term called hypersexuality. When this occurs, it is often due to the side effects of PD medications such as dopamine agonists or sometimes levodopa.

The following are factors that may contribute to sexual dysfunction:

- Psychological issues including depression, performance anxiety, and body image disturbance
- Atherosclerosis that may be caused by diabetes mellitus, high cholesterol, smoking, uncontrolled high blood pressure, and normal aging
- Endocrine disorders such as thyroid disease
- Hormone imbalance such as low levels of testosterone or estrogen
- Medications that decrease libido and/or cause impotence
- Parkinson's disease symptoms including rigidity, bradykinesia, and dyskinesia, which may affect mobility and manifest as fatigue, affecting stamina
- Concomitant depression in PD
- Side effects of other medications such as antidepressants (typically serotonin selective reuptake inhibitors [SSRIs]) that are commonly used in PD

As mentioned earlier, it is important to note that some Parkinson medications including carbidopa/levodopa and dopamine agonists may cause hypersexuality, an increased desire to have or think about sex.

Assessment

Many individuals are reluctant to discuss changes in sexual function with their health care provider and too often health care providers fail to assess if there is a problem.

A complete history and physical examination should be done to identify any problems with sexual function. Assessment should include evaluation of both physical and psychosocial causes. Referral to a urologist and for females to a gynecologist may be indicated.

Medications that contribute to sexual dysfunction should be identified. If indicated, thyroid function tests and hormone levels may need to be requested.

Nonpharmacological Management

- Provide a referral to a urologist specializing in male impotence as indicated.

- Provide a referral to a gynecologist for women experiencing decreased libido as indicated.
- Psychotherapy, family, or marriage counseling might help.
- Patients are instructed to use water-soluble lubricants (such as K-Y jelly) or estrogen creams.
- Share information with the patient on the importance of regular exercise and conditioning.

Pharmacological Management

- Optimize anti-Parkinson medication to provide symptom relief.
- Coordinate medication management with primary care physician to address concomitant medications that cause changes in sexual functioning.
- Treat depression; or change antidepressants from SSRIs to bupropion (Wellbutrin®).
- Prescribe medications that increase blood flow for erections including sildenafil (Viagra®), vardenafil (Levitra®), and tadalafil (Cialis®). These drugs lower blood pressure and should be used carefully. Also, if erection lasts longer than a few hours, seek medical attention immediately. Do not mix the medication with nitrates.
- When low hormonal levels are documented, hormonal therapy (such as testosterone replacement therapy) might help.

For patients with hypersexuality, lowering the dosage or eliminating the PD medication might alleviate the problem.

SHORTNESS OF BREATH

Individuals with Parkinson's disease may experience shortness of breath, also called dyspnea, related to the disease process and/or to treatment side effects.

Some causes include:

- Muscle rigidity of the chest wall and breathing musculature, causing less air movement in and out of the lungs and resulting in shortness of breath.
- Dyskinesia (involuntary movements), a motor complication of levodopa and dopamine agonists, which can be accompanied by shortness of breath (may be termed respiratory dyskinesia).

- Anxiety related to PD.
- The ergot dopamine agonists bromocriptine and pergolide. Individuals who have used the ergot dopamine agonists bromocriptine and pergolide are at risk of developing pulmonary complications from long-term use. Although rare, this should be considered when evaluating shortness of breath. Pergolide has been removed from the market and bromocriptine is rarely used.

Shortness of breath may be due to other health problems. Differential diagnosis includes:

- Emphysema, asthma
- Pulmonary embolus, pneumonia (including aspiration-related), inhalation of a foreign body
- Coronary artery disease, myocardial infarction
- Congestive heart failure (CHF), heart arrhythmias
- Deconditioning (lack of exercise)
- Obesity
- Panic attacks

Assessment

- Medical history and physical exam
- Referral to primary care provider for non-PD-related shortness of breath
- Blood tests including arterial blood gases
- Measurement of blood oxygen saturation (pulse oximetry)
- Electrocardiogram (ECG)
- X-ray of the chest
- Pulmonary function tests
- Exercise testing
- CT scan of the chest
- Echocardiogram

Pharmacological Management

- Optimize Parkinson disease medications as appropriate.
- Use anxiolytics to treat anxiety.

Nonpharmacological Management

- Provide referral to a physical therapist for strengthening, conditioning, range of motion (ROM), and breathing exercises.
- Use relaxation therapy to treat anxiety.

SLEEP PROBLEMS

Sleep disorders are common in Parkinson's disease and can greatly impact the quality of life of both the person with PD and the person's spouse or care provider. There are many reasons why sleep is disturbed, including the disease process, medication use, other health conditions, or normal aging. Usually there is more than one cause.

In normal aging, sleep patterns change. Duration of sleep often decreases and there are more interruptions during the night. In PD, sleep disorders can be divided into two main types: excessive daytime sleepiness and nighttime sleep disturbances.

In PD, sleep cycles become more fragmented. Individuals are usually able to fall asleep without difficulty but wake frequently during the night and have difficulty falling back to sleep. Sometimes, even after two or three hours, a person wakes and feels well rested as if a full night of sleep occurred. Many individuals report significant productivity during the night and early morning hours. Although positive, over time, the person feels unrested, often resulting in daytime sleepiness.

Changes in bladder function will often cause individuals with PD to develop increased urinary frequency at night. In addition people report an inability to move easily in bed and get comfortable. Most PD medications are used during the day when an individual requires dosing for improved mobility. A person may have increased rigidity at night and report difficulty moving in bed or turning in bed. PD medications are generally used sparingly at night to prevent insomnia. However, if discomfort from rigidity is present, then levodopa or dopamine agonists may be prescribed at bedtime.

Some individuals experience early-morning dystonia. Cramping, usually of the feet (toe curling) and legs, often described as a charley horse, disrupts sleep.

People with PD may also experience rapid eye movement (REM) behavior disorder as well as restless legs syndrome as described below.

REM Behavioral Sleep Disorder

REM behavioral sleep disorder (RBD) is characterized by the acting out of dreams that are vivid, intense, and violent. Some of these behaviors include talking, yelling, punching, kicking, sitting, jumping from bed, arm flailing, and grabbing. As a result individuals with RBD may injure themselves or their bed partner. The presence of RBD may precede the diagnosis of Parkinson's disease by many years or may occur after the disease has been diagnosed. A variety of medications, particularly antidepressants, may potentially worsen RBD. Diet and fatigue may also play a role. The diagnosis of RBD is usually made in the clinic, but often a confirmatory sleep study is useful to eliminate other possible diagnoses as well as determine if sleep apnea is also present. Treatment of RBD may include eliminating offending causative medications. Alternatively, a benzodiazepine compound such as clonazepam (Klonopin®) is used. Tolerance to the medication may occur and therefore the dose may be increased over time, and liver function tests may need to be monitored. A common side effect is sedation (to help the individual fall asleep), which can be prolonged and can cause a hangover type of grogginess the following day.

Restless Legs Syndrome

Restless legs syndrome (RLS) is a disorder that causes tingling, pulling, creeping, or painful sensations in the legs. Symptoms typically occur when lying down in bed, or when seated for prolonged periods such as while driving or at a theater. RLS typically occurs in the evening, making it difficult to fall asleep. Often, people with RLS have the urge to move their legs and as a result may get up and walk during the night. This restlessness and walking will affect sleep. RLS may be related to an iron deficiency, a genetic cause (familial RLS), peripheral neuropathy, radiculopathy, or a feature of PD.

Daytime Sleepiness

Sleepiness during the day is common with PD. A common cause for this is impaired sleep at night. The second factor may be PD medications (especially dopamine agonists and levodopa) or other medications that cause sleepiness. Third, sleepiness during the day may increase with aging as well as with the onset of dementia in some individuals. The presence of daytime sleepiness should be a warning for those who drive as they are probably at a higher risk for a motor vehicle accident. Improving sleep hygiene as well as reducing or eliminating sedating medications are the first steps. The addition of a stimulant medication such as methylphenidate (Ritalin®) or modafanil (Provigil®) is another option to manage the sleepiness.

Sleep Apnea

Although not directly related to PD, sleep apnea is a significant sleep disorder that occurs when a person's breathing is interrupted for over 15 seconds during sleep. People with untreated sleep apnea may stop breathing hundreds of times per night. In the long term this may be associated with cardiac or pulmonary disorders and even sudden death. Therefore, treatment of sleep apnea may reduce the risk of these issues. In order to evaluate for sleep apnea, a sleep study is needed that is usually preceded by a consultation with a sleep specialist. The sleep study evaluates for drops in blood oxygen levels caused by periods of apnea.

There are two types of sleep apnea: obstructive and central. Obstructive sleep apnea (OSA) is the more common of the two. There are some reports that this condition is overrepresented in PD compared to the general population. It is caused by a blockage of the airway, usually when the soft tissue in the rear of the throat collapses during sleep. OSA has been increasing along with obesity. Therefore, those individuals who are overweight and/or with enlarged or large necks are at risk for OSA. Meanwhile with central sleep apnea, the airway is not blocked but the brain fails to signal the muscles to breathe because of instability in the respiratory control center. This type is called central apnea because it is related to the function of the central nervous system.

Assessment

- Obtain the patient's sleep history from both the patient and family. Obtaining a sleep diary that has been kept for two weeks is helpful. Information in the diary should include hours asleep, waking times, and cause of waking if known.
- Some sleep scales have been developed that are useful in highlighting a patient's experience with sleep. These include the Epworth Sleep Scale and the Parkinson Disease Sleep Scale.
- Assess for presence of depression.

- Identify coexisting conditions contributing to sleep disturbance and treat as needed.
- When RLS is seen, it is often part of PD, but sometimes, a check on kidney function and iron-deficiency anemia may be needed, that is, obtain CBC, ferritin, creatinine, BUN, and so on.
- Ultimately, when a sleep disorder is strongly suspected, referral to a sleep specialist for a sleep study and evaluation may be needed. Polysomnography may catch sleep problems that are missed by histories and sleep diaries.
- A sleep study or polysomnogram (PSG) is a multiple-component test that electronically transmits and records specific physical activities during sleep. The recordings become data that are analyzed by a qualified physician to determine presence and/or cause of sleep disturbance.

Nonpharmacological Management

Patient and family education to review practices to improve quantity and quality of sleep include:

- Practice good sleep hygiene.
- Maintain a regular sleep schedule 7 days a week. Keep the same bedtime each night.
- Make the sleep environment as comfortable as possible. Consider a bed with capability to elevate head. Use satin sheets to move more easily. Install a grab bar or mobility-transfer handle to assist with turning and getting in and out of bed. Have a comfortable recliner chair in the room. Keep the bedroom clear of clutter.
- Avoid ingesting stimulants, including caffeine, nicotine, and alcohol, too close to bedtime.
- Participate in an active exercise program during the day.
- Spend part of the day outdoors, increasing natural exposure to light.
- Avoid heavy meals within 4 hours of bedtime.
- Limit fluid intake 4 hours before bedtime.
- Review Parkinson and concomitant medications with health care provider to determine if they interfere with sleep. Review optimal schedule with health care provider.

For individuals with REM sleep disorder, maintaining a safe sleep environment is paramount.

- Remove furniture or objects that could injure the person if he or she fell out of bed.
- Use padded side rails or a mattress close to the floor as needed.
- Encourage bed partner to use a separate bed during sleep time.

Sleep apnea is treated with weight reduction and the use of continuous positive airway pressure (CPAP), a treatment that uses slightly pressurized air throughout the breathing cycle. This makes it easier to breathe and get more air. CPAP can be used by mouth, by nose, or through ventilation tubes. Occasionally, surgery or other measures may be needed.

Pharmacological Management

There are many medications used to treat sleep disturbance. Different agents are used depending on the actual sleep problem. Most sleep medications have side effects and lose effectiveness over time. Therefore, sleep medications should be used sparingly.

Three over-the-counter medications include:

- Diphenhydramine (Benadryl®)
- Acetaminophen/diphenhydramine (Tylenol® PM; which contains benadryl)
- Melatonin

Prescription sleep medication includes:

- Zolpidem (Ambien®)
- Zaleplon (Sonata®)

Some antidepressants, anxiolytics, and antipsychotic medications have an added benefit of improving sleep and are sometimes used.

- Nortryptyline (Pamelor®)
- Trazodone (Desyrel®)
- Quetiapine (Seroquel®)
- Lorazepam (Ativan®)
- Clonazepam (Klonopin®)

Clonazepam (Klonopin®) is highly effective in the treatment of REM sleep behavior disorder (RBD), relieving symptoms in nearly 90%

of patients. However, there is always a risk of tolerance developing as well as, albeit usually low, a potential risk for abuse. The response usually begins within the first week, often on the first night. With continued treatment for years, moderate limb twitching with sleep talking and more complex behaviors can reemerge. The treatment should be continued indefinitely, as violent behaviors and nightmares promptly recur with discontinuation of medications in almost all persons with RBD.

Daytime sleepiness is treated by the use of stimulating medications. Modafanil (Provigil®) seems to have fewer side effects than traditional stimulants. It is FDA-approved for narcolepsy and may soon be approved for shift-work sleep disorder.

Restless legs syndrome in Parkinson's disease is treated by treating the underlying disorder and by treatment with dopamine agonists.

SOCIAL ISOLATION

Humans are social beings. Time spent with others gives meaning to life. When individuals are faced with the challenges of Parkinson's disease, social interactions are oftentimes disrupted. For the patient, physical changes such as a decreased facial expression or a muffled voice can result in cues that are misunderstood or misinterpreted by social contacts. For the caregiver and family, alterations in the ability to mingle with a social network in the same manner as before the PD diagnosis can result in disrupted socialization. Hence, social isolation affecting both the patient and the family is oftentimes a direct result of the physical and emotional demands of the illness. Individuals who are unable or do not want to leave the home due to decreased mobility, changes in cognitive status, depression, or embarrassment from symptoms are particularly at risk for social isolation. Health care providers play an important role in assessing the impact of Parkinson's on an individual and family's ability to socialize.

Assessment

Health care providers should directly ask the patient and family caregivers if they have experienced a decrease in socialization. Special attention should focus on:

- Patient's ability to communicate and be understood
- A change in number of social contacts

- Signs and symptoms of depression
- Means of transportation
- Availability of a support network and resources

Management

- Provide referral to a mental health provider including a psychologist and/or licensed social worker for counseling and support.
- Treat depression as indicated.
- Provide referral to a PD support group. In addition to receiving information on living with PD, individuals and families benefit from the social aspect of the group.
- Provide information and referral to supportive services including local Council on Aging services, community senior centers, Parkinson lay organizations, adult day health programs, and transportation services.
- Inform family members and direct care providers that individuals with Parkinson's disease may be slow to respond to questions or participate in conversation. Provide reassurance that the person understands exactly what is being said. An increased awareness of this and some patience will enhance communication.

SPEECH PROBLEMS

Speech problems in Parkinson's disease are both complex and multifactorial. Individuals may have difficulty with phonation, resonance, voice pitch, and articulation. Difficulty with speech impairs communication both at work and at home and affects a person's quality of life.

Phonation problems include a soft voice, or hypophonia. Interestingly people with PD often report that their voice volume seems normal when the low volume makes it difficult for others to hear. This lack of recognition not only impacts interpersonal relationships but also decreases the likelihood that a person will seek evaluation and treatment.

The resonance quality of voice is often hypernasal. Speech can be monotone with little inflection. Some individuals experience *pallilalia,* a constant repetition of syllables. In addition a person may have a festinating speech pattern, that is, a rapid rhythm with decreased enunciation of words. These two conditions are frustrating for both the person and family.

An altered voice arises from rigidity, slowness (bradykinesia), and less often tremor of the muscles of speech production. If chest-wall muscles become rigid, less air moves in and out of the lungs, which lessens the airflow to generate voice and as a result the voice is softer. Therapists describe this as having a lack of breath support. Individuals are taught to learn to breathe slowly and deeply, training the voice like an opera singer. It is necessary to generate enough air when speaking and to speak in shorter phrases.

Slurring of speech, also known as *dysarthria*, can occur with Parkinson's disease over time. Its appearance early on in the course of the condition may herald other Parkinson conditions including multiple system atrophy (MSA) or progressive supranuclear palsy (PSP).

Mild cognitive changes associated with PD can also affect an individual's linguistic ability. People often describe knowing what they want to say but having difficulty identifying or expressing a word or phrase. This difficulty coupled with slowness in response time significantly impairs the flow of conversation.

Assessment

Individuals with PD should be assessed for the presence of a speech and communication disorder by their health care providers throughout the course of the disease. The patient and family should be asked to describe any problems with speech or communication. The Unified Parkinson's Rating Scale (UPDRS) includes the following two items on speech that are useful for a quick assessment.

Impact on Activities of Daily Living

0 = Normal

1 = Mildly affected

2 = Moderately affected

3 = Severely affected

4 = Unintelligible most of the time

Motor Examination

0 = Normal

1 = Slight loss of expression

2 = Monotone, slurred but understandable; moderately impaired

3 = Marked impairment, difficult to understand

4 = Unintelligible

The impact of anti-Parkinson medications on speech is not completely understood; it is known that fluctuations in speech patterns can occur with fluctuations in dose and motor response. It may be useful for patients and families to document whether and how speech patterns change throughout the day.

A multidisciplinary approach to care includes collaboration with neurology, speech and language pathology, otolaryngology, and occupational therapy. Initial referral should be made to a speech and language pathologist experienced in the evaluation and treatment of Parkinson's disease. A complete evaluation of speech, hearing, and other factors associated with communication is performed. As with all rehabilitation therapies, early intervention is best. The speech and language pathologist may recommend referral to otolaryngology where an ear, nose, and throat (ENT) physician will provide evaluation of the larynx and vocal chords to rule out other problems that may contribute to speech disorders. Laryngoscopy may be performed. Barium swallow ultrasound is performed if voice changes are accompanied by swallowing difficulties.

Management

- The main treatment of communication problems (hypophonia and decreased articulation) involves the use of a specialized voice therapy treatment method called Lee Silverman Voice Treatment (LSVT). Prior to LSVT, speech therapy for Parkinson's disease patients had very little success. Research has shown significant improvement in quality of life, speech, and vocal function following the LSVT program. This intensive program is administered by a speech and language pathologist who has received specialized training.
- Voice amplification devices may be recommended for some individuals. These devices increase the loudness of speech but do not change the quality of speech. There are several commercial products available.

An otolaryngologist may perform a surgical intervention that can enhance voice volume. Medialization laryngoplasty or injection laryngoplasty with collagen is used to bulk up the weakened vocal folds. Not all individuals respond to this treatment.

- For most individuals with PD, pharmacological treatment does not appear to have a significant beneficial impact on speech production.
- Hyperkinetic dysarthria, often in the presence of dyskinesias after prolonged levodopa therapy, may also be encountered.
- Surgical treatments for PD do not have consistent significant benefit for the communication impairments associated with PD.

Patient/Family Educational Resources

Johnson, M. L. (2005). *Parkinson disease: Speech and swallowing* (2nd ed.). Miami, FL: National Parkinson Foundation.

Ruddy, B. H., & Sapienza, C. (2003). *Speaking effectively: A strategic guide for speaking and swallowing.* New York: American Parkinson Disease Association.

Health Care Professional Resources

1 Lee Silverman Voice Treatment Web site
www.lsvt.org

2 American Speech-Language-Hearing Association
www.asha.org
2200 Research Blvd.
Rockville, MD 20850-3289

SWALLOWING PROBLEMS

Although most people with Parkinson's disease will continue to eat normally throughout the course of the disease, some will develop difficulty with swallowing, called *dysphagia.* The severity of dysphagia may not correspond to the duration of PD or the severity of other motor symptoms. Swallowing problems in PD may include:

- Difficulty controlling the rate of food or liquid intake (e.g., eating food too quickly or impulsively, or eating very slowly due to difficulty handling food and bradykinesia)

- Difficulty chewing food
- Pocketing of food in the mouth
- Difficulty initiating a swallow
- Inability to swallow, or to complete a swallow

Complications of dysphagia include:

- Altered nutritional status, weight loss, and/or dehydration
- Risk of aspiration pneumonia
- Embarrassment when eating in a social setting
- Decrease in quality of life related to a decrease in the pleasure of eating

Although dysphagia is common in PD, it rarely is severe enough to require an alternative means of nutritional support. However, *gastrostomy* may be considered for some patients as an efficient means to provide additional nutritional support. In some situations, oral intake may continue with the presence of a gastrostomy tube.

Assessment

A swallowing evaluation is completed by a speech and language pathologist (SLP) who specializes in dysphagia.

- Obtain a history of disease process and symptoms (motor symptoms and cognition).
- Assess musculature involved in swallowing.
- Observe feeding patterns including rate of food intake, ability to chew, holding food or liquid in mouth, and ability to initiate a swallow.

Studies that may be performed include:

- Endoscopic assessment
- Modified barium swallow

Nonpharmacological Management

- Provide a referral to a speech and language pathologist to learn exercises to improve muscle movement and proper positioning for more effective swallowing.

- Alter food and liquid textures so that they are easier and safer to swallow. Use agents to thicken liquids. Choking is most common with thin liquids. Adding a thickening agent is helpful.
- The patient should sit upright at a 90-degree angle when eating.
- Provide adequate time for the patient to eat.
- Instruct patient and family to cut food into small pieces.
- Remind patients to swallow twice after each bite.
- Instruct the patient to alternate small bites and small sips in order to clear the food from the mouth.
- Teach the patient the chin down (also known as the chin tuck) technique, which is in actuality an attempt to keep the individual from aspirating food, which may occur if they extend their neck while swallowing. With this method, the patient should have his or her chin parallel to the table and not too far down as to cause food to fall out of his or her mouth or to make chewing and swallowing difficult. People with PD should raise their neck so their eyes look 30° above the horizon. They should sit with their elbows on the table, which automatically raises the chin and helps chewing and swallowing.
- Remind the patient and family caregiver to avoid foods such as raw vegetables, nuts, popcorn, and peanut butter that may be difficult to swallow.
- Advise patients to use easy-grip utensils to make feeding easier.
- Encourage the patient to practice good oral hygiene after meals, especially to remove all food particles from the mouth.
- Provide a referral to an occupational therapist qualified to assess feeding ability and recommend adaptive equipment that will promote independence with feeding.

Pharmacological Management

- Optimize Parkinson medications to decrease rigidity and improve fine-motor movement.
- Take levodopa preparations 30–60 minutes before meals to improve motor symptoms at meal time.

TREMOR

Tremor is one of the cardinal features of Parkinson's disease. This motor manifestation has been identified as a "resting tremor." When it occurs in the hand(s), it can also be described as "pill rolling" (i.e., a to-and-fro rhythmical movement between the thumb and forefinger). Like other motor symptoms associated with PD, it often starts unilaterally but typically progresses to also involve the other side of the body. Tremor most often affects the extremities but can also occur in the face, lips, and tongue. Some patients also state that they have an internal tremor or feeling of restlessness inside their bodies. Up to 30% of PD individuals may not experience any tremor. A small number of individuals will also have an action or postural tremor that increases with activity or change in position.

Severity of tremor fluctuates during the day. Excitement, stress, and even just being outside of the home (e.g., grocery store) may bring out tremor and/or increase the amplitude of an existing tremor. Tremor is thought to be the least disabling of the motor symptoms; however, its presence can cause fatigue as well as social embarrassment.

Assessment

- Medical history and physical examination are completed to differentiate PD tremor from other types of tremor (e.g., essential tremor). A careful family history is recorded, as 50% of individuals with tremor report one or more family members with a similar problem.
- The UPDRS includes three items on tremor. In *Part II—Activities of Daily Living,* patients are asked to rate their tremor as:

  0 = Absent

  1 = Slight and infrequently present

  2 = Moderate and bothersome to patient

  3 = Severe, interferes with many activities

  4 = Marked, interferes with most activities

In *Part III of the Motor Examination,* raters measure tremor at rest; of the face, lips, and chin; of the right and left hand and foot; as well as action or postural tremor of the hands.

Tremor at Rest

0 = Absent

1 = Slight and infrequently present

2 = Mild in amplitude and persistent or moderate in amplitude, but only intermittently present

3 = Moderate in amplitude and present more of the time

4 = Marked in amplitude and present more of the time

Action or Postural Tremor of Hands (using finger-to-nose test and extension of arms out in front of the person):

0 = Absent

1 = Slight, present with action

2 = Moderate in amplitude, present with action

3 = Moderate in amplitude, with posture holding as well as action

4 = Marked in amplitude, interferes with feeding

- A psychosocial assessment of the impact of tremor should be done including discussion on how bothersome tremor is for the person experiencing it. Is the tremor embarrassing? Has it affected socialization, employment, or relationships?

Pharmacological Management

- The decision on when to use pharmacological therapies to treat tremor should be individualized for each patient. This will depend on the type, severity, and impact of tremor on functional status and quality of life. Since anti-Parkinson medications are used to treat tremor, other considerations include the age and overall patient health as well as a concern for the development of motor complications.
- Pharmacologic response to tremor is variable from person to person.
- Initial low-dose therapy with a dopamine agonist and/or levodopa is the treatment of choice and may be increased for worsening of tremor.
- Anticholinergic therapies, including trihexyphenidyl (Artane®) or benztropine (Cogentin®), are used to treat tremor. They should be avoided in individuals who are elderly or are at risk of increased confusion due to the common side effects of confusion, urinary retention, blurred vision, and dry mouth.

- Amantadine may be used for mild tremor.
- Primidone or propranolol is sometimes prescribed to treat action or postural tremors.

Nonpharmacological Management

- Provide a referral to an occupational therapist to identify strategies to improve function with tremor. For example, using a special computer mouse for easy navigation may be helpful for some patients.
- Provide referral to a mental health provider if tremor is impacting coping abilities. Some individuals benefit from using relaxation techniques during times of increased tremor.
- Deep brain stimulation is used for moderate to severe tremor that responds poorly to medication and that significantly impacts quality of life. Candidates for DBS should be carefully screened for appropriateness for surgery.

URINARY DYSFUNCTION

In Parkinson's disease there are difficulties with bladder control duc to nervous system changes that regulate bladder function. In PD the bladder becomes overactive and may suddenly contract, resulting in urinary urgency and increased frequency of urination. The volume of urine produced at each void is often less than typically occurs. These features may be present during the day or at night (nocturia) with the latter resulting in disrupted sleep. In addition individuals may also experience impairment of bladder emptying, often due to a coexisting condition such as an enlarged prostate in men. These individuals report hesitancy in urination and difficulty generating a stream of urine. Coexisting conditions causing urinary dysfunction should be considered when developing a plan of care. Medications used to treat one condition may actually worsen another condition.

Potential Causes of Urinary Changes

- Parkinson's disease
- Other age-related urinary tract changes
- Enlarged prostate in men, which complicates urinary flow

- In women, weakness in the muscles of the pelvis that develops as they age
- Certain over-the-counter and prescription medications that can make bladder control problems worse

Assessment

A careful medical history should be done to note voiding frequency, urgency, volume, incontinence, and a history of urinary infections. Information should also be obtained regarding the patient's ability to toilet independently.

Referral to a urologist may be necessary to evaluate urinary dysfunction. Diagnostic tests that may be performed include:

- Urinalysis
- Urine culture to check for infection if indicated
- Cystoscopy
- Urodynamic studies (to measure pressure and urine flow)
- Uroflow (to measure pattern of urine flow)
- Post-void residual (PVR) to measure amount of urine left in the bladder immediately following micturation

Other tests may be performed to rule out pelvic weakness as the cause of the incontinence. One such test is called the Q-tip test. This test involves measurement of the change in the angle of the urethra when it is at rest and when it is straining. An angle change of greater than 30° often indicates significant weakness of the muscles and tendons that support the bladder.

Nonpharmacological Management

Patient and family teaching includes information on:

- Pelvic floor muscle exercises (Kegel exercises). These exercises can strengthen the muscles that help hold urine inside the bladder. How does one do these exercises?

    1. Pull in or tighten pelvic muscles and hold for a count of 3.
    2. Then completely relax the muscle for a count of 3.

3. Repeat 10–15 times, at least 3 times per day.
4. Each time you do these exercises, alternate your position between lying, sitting, and standing.

- Bladder retraining:

  1. Schedule bathroom trips. Begin every 2 hours while awake and work up to every 4 hours between trips.
  2. Suppress the urge to void:
     - a. Take slow, deep breaths through your mouth, concentrating on breathing.
     - b. Tighten pelvic floor muscle quickly, several times in a row.
     - c. Concentrate on suppressing the need to void.
  3. Use a bladder diary to monitor success.

Patient and family caregivers should be advised to:

- Limit intake of fluids after 6:00 P.M.
- Use grab bars and adequate lighting in the bathroom to improve mobility and safety.
- Use a bedside commode or urinal to ease the difficulty of getting to and from the bathroom during the night.
- Use incontinence aids including pads. Share information with the patient and family about how to use and apply incontinence aids including the use of a condom catheter for men.

Pharmacological Management

Bladder medications commonly used to decrease urinary frequency, urgency, or incontinence include oxybutynin (Ditropan®, Oxytrol®), tolterodine tartrate (Detrol®), solifenacin (Vesicare®), and darifenacin (Enablex®). They work by relaxing the bladder muscle and reducing involuntary contractions.

1. Oxybutynin (Ditropan®, Oxytrol®)
   - a. Dosing
     - The usual oral dose of immediate-release oxybutynin for adults is 5 mg, 2 or 3 times daily with a maximum of 5 mg, 4 times daily.
     - The recommended starting dose of extended release oxybutynin is 5 or 10 mg once daily at approximately the same time

of day. Dosage may be increased in 5 mg increments at approximately weekly intervals to a maximum of 30 mg daily.

b Side effects: The following side effects can occur with the use of oxybutynin:

- Dry mouth
- Sensitivity to bright light
- Blurred vision
- Dry eyes
- Decreased sweating
- Flushing
- Nausea
- Drowsiness
- Confusion

2 Tolterodine tartrate (Detrol®)

a Dosing

- The initial recommended dose of immediate-release tolterodine is 2 mg orally twice daily; may decrease to 1 mg twice daily depending on tolerability and response.
- The initial recommended dose of extended-release tolterodine is 4 mg orally once daily; may decrease to 2 mg once daily depending on tolerability and response.

b Side effects: The following side effects can occur with the use of tolterodine:

- Dry mouth
- Blurred vision
- Nausea
- Headache
- Constipation
- Dry eyes
- Dizziness

Solifenacin (Vesicare®) and darifenacin (Enablex®) are the newest medications used to treat an overactive bladder and urinary incontinence.

VISION PROBLEMS

Individuals with Parkinson's disease often report changes in vision. These are caused by aging because of changes in the lens, glaucoma, cataracts, and sometimes macular degeneration, combined with the loss of dopamine retinal cells and other PD symptoms. The cause, presentation, and treatment of each symptom or condition are multifactorial and require a comprehensive evaluation by an eye specialist.

1 Dry eyes
Bradykinesia decreases eye blinking. The tear film that keeps the eye moist dries out. In addition, some medications that are used in PD decrease tear secretion. The eyes subsequently become dry and irritated.

2 Double vision
In PD the ability to coordinate the movements of the two eyes together is impaired, sometimes resulting in double vision. It is usually intermittent and can respond to anti-Parkinson medications. It occurs most often with reading or close vision, and in the evening when the person is more tired.

Progressive supranuclear palsy (PSP) is a condition that includes many features of parkinsonism. Individuals with PSP have striking changes in eye movements that particularly affect downward gaze.

3 Blurred vision
A variety of medications may cause blurred vision. The anticholinergic drugs trihexyphenidyl (Artane®) and benztropine (Cogentin®), which are used sometimes to treat tremor in PD, are noteworthy for their potential to cause blurry vision. Likewise, other medications that also affect acetylcholine such as bladder medications (e.g., oxybutinin/Ditropan® and tolerodine/Detrol®) can cause this problem.

4 Blepharospasm
People with PD and other Parkinson conditions such as progressive supranuclear palsy (PSP) occasionally develop involuntary closure of the eyes, termed blepharospasm. At its mildest, there may be increased blinking; however, when more severe, there can be prolonged closure of the eyes and difficulty opening the eyes. More common than blepharospasm in PD is a condition called apraxia of eyelid opening. This is different from blepharospasm since the patient experiences difficulty opening the eyes instead of involuntary forceful closure of the eyes.

Blepharospasm or apraxia of eyelid opening in PD may be due to medications. If a relationship is found between the onset of the blepharospasm and a PD medication, it may be reasonable to try stopping the "offending" agent. Sometimes blepharospasm or apraxia of eyelid opening occur as part of motor fluctuations—either wearing off or diphasic dyskinesia—therefore, optimization of anti-PD medication may relieve this problem.

Nonetheless, stopping medications may not be easy, so the physician often resorts to the use of botulinum toxin injections to treat this problem. There are two forms of botulinum toxin: type A (also known as Botox®), and type B (which is Myobloc®), that can be used for injections into muscles around the eye (see Figure 1.4). The injections are administered with a small needle and there can be some temporary bruising. Benefit may start within a few hours to a week after the injection and the benefit may last between 1 and 6 months. One risk with the injections is for the potential further dryness of the eyes due to the desired reduction in blinking. Careful monitoring is needed including the use of artificial tear eyedrops throughout the day. This may be combined with ophthalmic lubricating ointment applied into the eyes at night along with taping the eyelid shut to keep the eyes from being open and drying out at night.

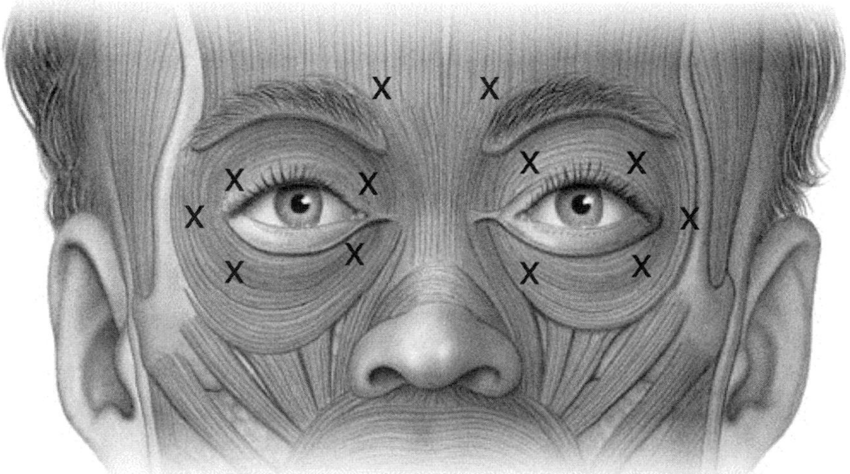

Figure 1.4 The typical location of botulinum toxin injections for blepharospasms and apraxia of eyelid opening.

5 Decreased contrast sensitivity
This is secondary to the loss of dopamine from retinal cells, and causes difficulty seeing contrasts, particularly when reading. More often, however, decrease in contrast sensitivity, depth perception, and color discrimination in PD is subtle and seen only with special tests.

Assessment

Provide a referral to an ophthalmologist for a complete eye examination and correction of refractive errors. This should be done annually. A neuro-ophthalmologist specializes in the impact of neurological conditions on vision.

Tests may include:

- Retinal examination
- Intraocular pressure measurement by tonometry
- Visual field assessment
- Visual acuity
- Refraction
- Pupillary reflex response
- Slit lamp examination
- Optic nerve imaging (photographs of the interior of the eye)
- Gonioscopy (use of a special lens to see the outflow channels of the angle)

Review medications used for Parkinson's disease and other conditions to identify agents that may affect vision.

Identify relationship of anti-Parkinson medication with presence of vision problem. For example, does double vision increase when Parkinson medications wear off?

Assess eye blink frequency and note presence of dry eyes. Individuals who have dry eyes often have excess tearing because the tear glands secrete when the eye is irritated.

Nonpharmacological Management

- For mild intermittent double vision, instruct the patient to close one eye. If the problem is more persistent, special glasses with prisms may be made for reading and other close activities.

- If reading is difficult for the patient, recommend using books on tape. A service of the National Library provides talking books. For information contact 1-888-657-7323.

Pharmacological Management

- Use artificial tears to improve symptoms. Preservative-free artificial tears can be used as often as needed. Artificial tears with preservatives should not be used more than every 2 hours. Multidose preparations must have preservatives. Single-dose preparations can be preservative-free but are usually more costly.

WALKING/GAIT ABNORMALITIES

Gait abnormalities in PD include reduced walking speed, shortened stride length, shuffling gait, impaired balance with a feeling of unsteadiness, festination (a tendency toward rapid forward movement), start hesitation, and gait freezing. These problems may increase disability, increase risk of injury, and also affect a person's quality of life.

Medications used to treat Parkinson symptoms may or may not improve an individual's gait. Evaluation of gait should take place when the patient is "on" as well as "off."

A multidisciplinary approach to the treatment of gait abnormalities includes referral to a physical therapist trained in the management of PD.

Assessment

- Medical history and physical examination to assess patterns of gait
- Assessment done in both the patient's "on" and "off" motor state
- Two-minute walk test and timed up-and-go test (TUG) to measure walking speed
- The Unified Parkinson Disease Rating Scale includes the following items related to walking:

Walking

0 = Normal

1 = Mild difficulty; may not swing arms or may tend to drag leg

2 = Moderate difficulty, but requires little or no assistance

3 = Severe disturbance of walking, requiring assistance

4 = Cannot walk at all, even with assistance

Freezing When Walking

1= None

2 = Rare freezing when walking, may have start hesitation

3 = Occasional freezing when walking

4 = Falls an average of once daily

5 = Falls more than once daily

Gait

0 = Normal

1 = Walks slowly, may shuffle with short steps, but no festination or propulsion

2 = Walks with difficulty, but requires little or no assistance; may have some festination, short steps, or propulsion

3 = Severe disturbance of gait, requiring assistance

4 = Cannot walk at all even with assistance

Nonpharmacological Management

Provide referral to a physical therapist who will participate in the following activities:

- Gait training to increase step length and overcome gait freezing
- Use of rhythmic auditory stimulation including music or metronome with specific beats to increase speed and quality of gait
- Use of visual stimulation techniques to interrupt gait freezing
  - Step over lines or follow a pattern on the floor
  - Step over a flashing light or steady beam of light (laser)
  - Look through, not directly at, doorways
- Teaching strategies to improve functional mobility: sit-to-stand, bed mobility

- Fall prevention and balance training
- Strengthening, range of motion, flexibility, and endurance training
- Assess need for assistive devices including a cane or walker

Patient/family education includes:

- Information on choosing footwear; improper shoes or heel height will affect gait, and high heels or rubber soles should be avoided
- The importance of maintaining good posture when sitting and standing
- Regular walking practice, including exaggerated lifting of feet and swinging the arms
- When turning, walking a circle instead of pivoting
- Noting relationship of walking difficulty with medication time and response, and sharing information with the health care provider
- Walking only with assistance if gait is unsteady
- Clearing walkways of clutter, removing throw rugs, and installing handrails as appropriate

Pharmacological Management

- Optimize Parkinson medications that improve gait disturbances

Available Resources

Where to buy a metronome:

- www.wwbw.com
- Free online metronome, http://www.metronomeonline.com
- Local music shop priced between $20 and $40

Assistive devices for gait:

- U Step™ walker or laser cane www.ustep.com
- NextStep™ cane www.icanstep.com

WEIGHT LOSS/GAIN

Weight changes may occur with Parkinson's disease. Typically a weight loss is observed but in certain circumstances a weight gain may occur.

Unplanned weight loss may lead to malnutrition, a significant health risk. Weight changes, whether losses or gains, usually occur over time. Conditions promoting weight change are multifactorial.

Weight loss may be attributed to:

- Changes in appetite due to decreased smell and diminished taste buds
- Immobility, making it difficult to access food and prepare adequate meals
- Difficulty chewing and swallowing foods
- Slow movement, making it difficult to finish meals on time
- Effects of medication, including nausea
- Presence of involuntary movements (dyskinesia), burning more calories
- Coexisting depression or dementia
- Medical conditions unrelated to Parkinson's disease (such as thyroid conditions, malignancy, and so forth)

Weight gain may be attributed to:

- Increased caloric intake due to obsessive eating, an adverse effect of dopaminergic medication
- A strong desire to eat sweets, including chocolate, ice cream, cakes, and cookies
- Decreased physical activity due to immobility
- Deep brain stimulation
- Medical conditions unrelated to Parkinson's disease

Assessment

To determine the causes of a change in weight, the following tests may be performed:

- Nutritional assessment
- Review body mass index, which is calculated based on height and weight; see Web sites http://www.nhlbisupport.com/bmi/ or http://www.cdc.gov/nccdphp/dnpa/healthyweight/assessing/bmi/index.htm
- Blood tests including chemistry profile
- Measurement of hormone levels

Table 1.4

ASSESSMENT FOR WEIGHT LOSS

TIME FRAME	SIGNIFICANT WEIGHT LOSS
1 week	Greater than or equal to 1%–2%
1 month	Greater than or equal to 5%
3 months	Greater than or equal to 7.5%
6 months	Greater than or equal to 10%

- Inventory of PD and non-PD medications
- Behavioral assessment to rule our depression or other behavioral conditions

Determination of an appropriate body weight for an individual is calculated by generating a number called the body mass index (BMI) that takes into account the individual's height along with their weight. Body weight is a good indicator of nutritional status. In addition, weight loss should always be evaluated for significance. This is done by calculating percent weight change and comparing it to the chart below.

1. $$\%\text{ weight change} = \frac{(\text{usual weight} - \text{current weight})}{\text{usual weight}} \times 100$$
2. Assessment for significant weight loss (see Table 1.4)

Nonpharmacological Management

For individuals experiencing a significant weight loss:

- Provide a referral to a nutritionist/registered dietitian (RD) to establish potential causes of weight loss and implement a well balanced diet.
- Instruct the patient to choose high-calorie foods, including prepared supplements.
- Instruct the patient to eat five small meals a day to conserve energy.

- Optimize PD medications to decrease adverse effects, including nausea and dyskinesia.
- Provide a referral to a speech and language pathologist for a speech and swallowing evaluation.

For individuals experiencing a significant weight gain:

- Provide a referral to a nutritionist to establish potential causes of weight gain and implement an appropriate well-balanced dietary plan to reduce weight.
- Provide a referral to a physical therapist to implement an exercise program.

Pharmacological Management

- Parkinson medication should be administered 30–60 minutes before meals to ensure optimal absorption and effect in time for meals.
- However, if significant nausea is experienced, PD medications may be taken *with meals* to minimize this side effect.
- For patients with weight gain of unclear etiology despite thorough assessment, tapering or discontinuing the dopamine agonist (such as ropinirole, pramipexole, or rotigotine) may be considered.

Patient/Family Educational Resources

Holden, K. (1998). *Eat well, stay well with Parkinson's disease.* Fort Collins, CO: Five Star Living. For patients and families. Copies may be ordered from Five Star Living, Inc., 1409 Olive Ct., Unit E, Fort Collins, CO 80524. Telephone: 877-565-2665.

Loew, J. E., & Pratt, C. (2007). *Good nutrition and Parkinson's disease.* New York: American Parkinson Disease Association.

Evaluation

SECTION II

This section will alphabetically include the various evaluations that an individual with Parkinson's disease may undergo or participate in during the course of his/her illness. Parkinson symptoms are highly variable from one patient to another. Evaluation and treatment must be individualized; therefore, not all of these evaluative procedures will apply to each patient.

GENETIC TESTING IN PARKINSON'S DISEASE

There have been significant advances in finding genetic causes for PD and to date several genes have been identified. However, these genetic forms are rare and the majority of individuals with PD do not carry one of the identified genes. It is for this reason that genetic testing is not done on a routine basis. It is usually performed if there is a strong family history, or in patients with young-onset PD. Only three genes can be commercially tested at this time: Parkin, Pink-1, and LRRK2. Information gained from this testing does not alter treatment at this point in time. There is ongoing study to determine if genetic information is useful in predicting long-term prognosis.

Genetic testing is expensive. The risks and benefits of testing should be discussed in detail by the patient and the health care provider.

IMAGING

Magnetic Resonance Imaging

Magnetic resonance imaging (MRI) of the brain is used in a Parkinson's disease evaluation to *rule out* other causes of parkinsonism including stroke, tumor, and infection. The results, however, will not confirm that a person has Parkinson's disease.

Another reason for obtaining an MRI is a sudden or unusual change in the patient's thinking, alertness, behavior, and motor control. Parkinson patients may also develop strokes and other neurological conditions unrelated to PD that can be detected with imaging.

This procedure takes approximately one hour to complete. Patients must lie still on the scanner table during the entire exam. Many people with PD have difficulty staying still. This is due to tremor, dyskinesia, or the uncomfortable feeling of muscle rigidity. Some individuals become very anxious. It is not unusual to have to abandon the test before completion. Patients who may have difficulty completing an MRI can be given a mild anxiolytic such as lorazepam.

Safety Concerns

- Metallic objects should not be allowed into the MRI scanning room.
- MRI should not be performed on individuals with implanted devices such as pacemakers, cochlear implants, brain aneurysm clips, some artificial heart valves, older vascular stents, and recently placed artificial joints. If there is any question, review the item with the radiology technician or/and radiologist.
- Patients with deep brain stimulation (DBS) should not have MRI unless the radiologist and neurologist agree that it is safe.
- Anyone who could have had shrapnel in them or exposure to other pieces of metal (such as sheet metal workers) should be screened before MRI.
- Occasionally, those with tattoos that contain metallic ink may have a warm uncomfortable feeling from the effects of the MRI on the tattoo.

Evaluation

Patients should be notified of MRI results in a timely manner even if the results are normal.

Several studies are ongoing using fMRI (functional magnetic resonance imaging). It is a neuroimaging technique used to study the activity or function, rather than the anatomy, of the brain. It shows which structures are active during particular mental operations.

Two other types of imaging include PET scans (positron emission tomography) and SPECT (single photon emission computerized tomography) scans. These diagnostic scans are used to evaluate function of the basal ganglia. Studies are ongoing to evaluate their efficacy in differential diagnosis and determination of disease progression.

NEUROLOGICAL EVALUATION

Most individuals with Parkinson's disease will report their first symptoms to or often have their symptoms identified by a primary care physician. After the medical history is obtained and the physical examination is performed, the patient is often referred to a neurologist to confirm a diagnosis of PD. This may be a general neurologist or in some cases a movement disorder specialist (MDS), with special training in Parkinson's disease. Several factors influence the ability to see an MDS including: health care referral practices, availability of specialists in a geographical region, complexity of the case, and the desire of a patient to see a movement specialist. Patients who are not diagnosed or followed early in their disease process often seek consultation with an MDS as the disease progresses. It is not unusual for a patient to receive more than one opinion and sometimes several over the course of their illness.

Referral to an MDS or to a movement disorder center is important because:

- PD is complex; it has both primary and secondary symptoms that may affect all body systems.
- PD occurs in a population that, by virtue of its age, often has coexisting chronic disease(s).
- Treatment of both the PD and potential coexisting disease requires numerous medications.
- Timing of medication administration to treat PD symptoms is often more crucial than with other diseases.

- A comprehensive rehabilitation approach is needed to maintain mobility and treat symptoms not responsive to medication.
- The patient with PD and the patient's family require significant teaching to participate in managing the disease.
- The health care team is often multidisciplinary, requiring frequent detailed communications with primary care providers, speech and swallowing clinicians, physical and occupational therapists, and sometimes psychiatrists, psychologists, family counselors, nutritionists, and other specialists.
- Research is dynamic, providing new insights into established treatments and novel medications.

NEURO-OPHTHALMOLOGY CONSULTATION

Neuro-ophthalmology is a medical specialty that is concerned with neurological problems of the eye and vision. Physicians with this specialty have extensive training in both neurology and ophthalmology.

Eye problems in PD are often subtle and recognized only in formal eye testing. Therefore, some individuals with PD may need to be referred to a neuro-ophthalmologist if they are experiencing problems with double vision, blurred vision, decreased visual acuity, and changes in contrast sensitivity resulting from dysfunction of dopamine receptors in the retina. Other eye problems managed by the neuro-ophthalmologist include dry eyes and excessive tearing resulting from a decrease in eye blink, as well as blepharospasm, an involuntary closure of the eyes.

Evaluation may include:

- Examination of the eye orbit, the eyelids, and the degree of opening (i.e., palpebral fissure)
- Pupillary evaluation to examine size, shape, and reactivity of the pupils to light and dark
- Visual acuity and color vision testing
- Visual field testing to look for areas of visual loss, which may include Amsler grid, Goldman perimetry
- Examination of the fundus, retina, and optic disk
- Assessment of extraocular eye muscle movements

Some patients experience visual hallucinations (seeing things that aren't there) or have illusions (misinterpreting visual stimuli). It is important to eliminate ophthalmologic causes before concluding that it may be due to PD medications or possibly associated with cognitive changes.

When involuntary/forceful closure of the eyelids (termed *blepharospasm*) or difficulty with voluntary opening of the eyes (termed *apraxia of eyelid opening*) occur, treatment with botulinum toxin injection may be considered. This is usually performed by a neuro-ophthalmologist or a neurologist specializing in Parkinson's disease.

NEUROPHYSIOLOGICAL STUDIES

Neurophysiological studies include electroencephalogram (EEG), electromyography (EMG), sleep studies, and autonomic testing. EEG and EMG are typically not useful in the diagnosis of Parkinson's disease but may be ordered to rule out other conditions.

An EEG records the electrical activity of the brain via surface electrodes applied to the scalp. It is a painless procedure and is used to diagnose seizures and toxic, metabolic, and infectious encephalopathies. An EMG records the conduction of peripheral nerves and the activity of muscles. It is performed when a peripheral neuropathy, radiculopathy, or myopathy are suspected. This procedure can sometimes be uncomfortable, but the pain or discomfort is often tolerable.

Sleep studies are useful in Parkinson's disease because of the high incidence of sleep disorders. Almost all PD patients will have some form of sleep disturbance: difficulty falling asleep at night, fragmented night sleep, or excessive daytime sleepiness. These studies are performed overnight in a sleep laboratory. Electrodes are applied to the scalp and limbs. Results are used to diagnose various disorders that could be associated with PD including sleep apnea, REM sleep behavior disorder, restless legs syndrome, and nocturnal myoclonus (also called *periodic leg movements of sleep*).

Autonomic studies evaluate the function of the autonomic nervous system, which is often affected in Parkinson's disease. Autonomic symptoms include constipation, urinary dysfunction, excessive sweating, and orthostatic hypotension. Autonomic studies are performed in a specially equipped laboratory and are indicated in patients with suspected orthostatic hypotension. They may help differentiate idiopathic Parkinson's disease from multiple system atrophy (MSA). Testing includes having the patient lie on a tilt table. Blood pressure and electrocardiogram are recorded as the table is tilted upright.

NEUROPSYCHOLOGICAL EVALUATION

Neuropsychological testing is performed to evaluate changes in mood, behavior, memory, and concentration that may occur in Parkinson's disease. In PD the fronto-subcortical areas of the brain (responsible for analytical thinking and processing of complex tasks) are most affected; however, significant research is ongoing to understand the impact PD has on other areas. There is interest in identifying neuropsychological changes in individuals at risk for developing dementia. Reasons to refer a PD patient to a neuropsychologist include:

- Assessment and etiology of changes in cognition (e.g., depression, strokes, medication, etc.)
- Evaluation to rule out dementia or depression prior to deep brain stimulation surgery
- Evaluation of the effect of pharmacological agents used to treat changes in cognition (i.e., cholinesterase inhibitors)

Individuals referred for neuropsychological testing should be informed on what to expect and how to prepare for it. This will help alleviate the anxiety that patients and families often experience before and during testing. Generally the neuropsychologist will begin the session with an interview. This is followed by the administration of a series of tests usually administered by a technician. A complete review of all test results is done by the neuropsychologist and a report is prepared and sent to the referring health care provider. This comprehensive report summarizes test results, observations, impressions, and recommendations.

Helpful tips to prepare a patient for neuropsychological testing include:

- Scheduling testing early in the day and at a time when the patient best responds to PD medication and has the best function
- Instructing the patient, if applicable, to wear eyeglasses and their hearing aid during testing
- Reminding the patient to bring all medications and take them as usual during the session
- Informing the patient and family caregiver that the tests are long and sometimes difficult; emphasizing that this is a common experience of all people who participate in this testing and that no one is expected to answer all questions correctly

Patients should answer all the questions regarding their behavior as truthfully as they can. They should not try to second-guess or anticipate the correct answer. The best answer is how they honestly feel.

NUTRITIONAL CONSULTATION

Nutritional consultation with a registered dietician (RD) is recommended for all patients with Parkinson's disease. Ideally the nutritionist should have a working understanding of the nutritional concerns of PD.

Patients are at risk for an altered nutritional status because of:

- Swallowing difficulties, slow feeding, and chewing
- Inability to prepare meals
- Weight loss or weight gain
- Bone loss or osteoporosis
- Constipation
- Vitamin deficiency

Nutritional assessment will include:

- Health history
- Current medication, vitamin, mineral, and supplement use
- Physical examination; weight, body mass index (BMI)
- Laboratory tests (such as levels of electrolytes, vitamins, and minerals, and dual energy X-ray absorptiometry [DEXAscan])
- Current behaviors and attitudes associated with eating
- Bowel habits, for example, constipation
- Relationship of levodopa response to protein and fat intake
- Three-day food and medication diary

Patients may require counseling on the use of vitamins and minerals. Some patients experience a lack of efficacy of a levodopa dose when they take it with foods high in protein and fats. Patients are instructed on medication timing, dietary choices, and protein redistribution. Additional instruction of food choices, including the use of increased fiber and water to alleviate constipation, are made. Other dietary discussions includes the importance of following a well-balanced diet. Although reasons are unclear, many individuals with PD have an increased desire to eat sweets, including ice cream and chocolate. Some of these may be side effects of certain medications.

Patient Education

Holden, K. (1998). *Eat well, stay well with Parkinson's disease.* Fort Collins, CO: Five Star Living. For patients and families. Copies may be ordered from Five Star Living, Inc., 1409 Olive Ct., Unit E, Fort Collins, CO 80524. Telephone: 877-565-2665.

Holden, K. (2000). *Parkinson's disease and constipation.* Fort Collins, CO: Five Star Living. Audiotape and guidebook for patients, families, and group use. Available from Five Star Living, Inc., 1409 Olive Ct. Unit E, Fort Collins, CO 80524. Telephone: 877-565-2665.

PARKINSON'S DISEASE RATING SCALES

Parkinson's disease is a complex medical condition that can affect an individual's physical, mental, and social well-being. The disease is slowly progressive over several years, highly individualized, and often difficult to characterize. Several rating scales have been developed to measure the impact of PD on a patient and family. These scales are used primarily in research to:

- Determine eligibility to participate in a research trial
- Assess severity and disease progression

Scales may also be used in clinical practice to:

- Identify and monitor problems in clinical practice
- Gauge clinical function and degree of disease progression

Scales currently in use have been developed or modified specifically for Parkinson's disease, evaluated for reliability and validity, and updated to measure new phenomenology. It is important to note that perfecting assessment tools is always a work in progress.

Scales Specific to Parkinson's Disease

1 Unified Parkinson Disease Rating Scale (UPDRS)
   - The UPDRS is a scale designed to monitor Parkinson's disease (PD) disability and impairment. It is the most commonly used

clinical scale for the evaluation of parkinsonian motor impairment and disability in published treatment trials.

- The scale has four sections
  - Part I Mentation, behavior, and mood
  - Part II Activities of daily living
  - Part III Motor examination
  - Part IV Complications of therapy
- Part I examines for intellectual impairment, thought disorders, depression, and changes in motivation/initiative. Part II includes 13 items of activities of daily living. Part III evaluates motor impairment including speech, facial expression, rest and postural tremor, rigidity, bradykinesia, posture, gait, and postural stability. Part IV addresses complications of therapy including dyskinesias, clinical fluctuations, and other complications.

2 Modified Hoehn and Yahr Scale

- This scale provides a global assessment of severity in PD based on clinical findings and functional disability.
- Originally, the scale comprised a five-point system:
  - Stage I. Unilateral involvement only, usually with minimal or no functional impairment.
  - Stage II. Bilateral or midline involvement, without impairment of balance.
  - Stage III. Bilateral involvement with balance changes, for example, impaired righting reflexes. Functionally, the patient is somewhat restricted in his activities but may have some work potential, depending upon the type of employment. Patients are physically capable of leading independent lives, and their disability is mild to moderate.
  - Stage IV. Fully developed, severely disabling disease; the patient is still able to walk and stand unassisted but is markedly incapacitated.
  - Stage V. Confinement to bed or wheelchair unless aided.
- The Modified Hoehn and Yahr has half-point increments (1.0, 1.5, 2.0, 2.5, 3.0, 4.0, 5.0).

3 Schwab and England Disability Scale

- This is a 100-point disability scale, with 10-point decrements from complete independence (100%) to complete dependence (0%).
- This scale has been extensively used as a standard instrument in PD studies, and is often tagged with the UPDRS.

4 Abnormal Involuntary Movement Scale (AIMS)
- This is a 12-item instrument originally developed to assess abnormal involuntary movements in psychiatric patients.
- The severity of any involuntary movement (excluding tremor) is scored on a 5-point scale (0 = none, 4 = severe) in the various anatomic regions.
- The scale includes a global judgment section with two questions directed towards the examiner (severity of abnormal movements, incapacitation due to abnormal movements), and one towards the patient (awareness of abnormal movements).
- It is most commonly used to assess tardive dyskinesia (drug-induced involuntary movements that are seen after about 6 months of being on a medication). In patients with PD, the AIMS is used to assess the severity of levodopa-induced dyskinesias.

Quality of Life Assessment in PD

1 PDQUALIF
- This is a 33-item instrument that includes seven domains: social/role function, self-image/sexuality, sleep, outlook, physical function, independence, and urinary function.
- The scale includes one item on the global quality of life.
- The PDQUALIF has been used in several clinical trials in PD.

2 PDQ39
- This is a disease-specific measure of subjective health status that is completed by patients.
- There are 39 items on the questionnaire, and scores indicate the impact of PD over the past month in eight dimensions of health status:
  - Mobility, 10 items
  - Activities of daily living, 6 items
  - Emotional well-being, 6 items
  - Stigma, 4 items
  - Social support, 3 items
  - Cognitions, 4 items
  - Communication, 3 items
  - Bodily discomfort, 3 items
- Each item can be scored as 0 (never impacts), 1 (rarely impacts), 2 (sometimes impacts), 3 (often impacts), or 4 (always impacts).

- In addition, a global index score, the PD Summary Index (PDSI), gives an overall idea of the impact of PD on health status.
- A reduced size questionnaire (PDQ8) shows reasonable correlation with PDQ39.

Cognitive Assessment in PD

1 Mini Mental Status Exam (MMSE)
- This is a standardized and validated scale used as a screening instrument for cognitive impairment.
- It measures the following cognitive domains:
  - Orientation
  - Registration and short-term recall
  - Concentration/attention
  - Verbal language (naming, repetition, following three-step commands)
  - Written language (reading and writing)
  - Visuospatial function (constructing a diagram)
- The MMSE is scored using a 30-point scale:
  - Scores in a range of 26–30 are generally considered normal in the general population.
  - Scores between 24 and 26 are considered questionable or indicative of very mild impairment.
  - Scores below 24 are abnormal, with 21–24 indicating mild cognitive impairment, 10–20 indicating moderate cognitive impairment, and <10 indicating severe impairment.
- While this is perhaps the most popular cognitive screening test, it may not be very sensitive to early cognitive impairment in PD.

2 Montreal Cognitive Assessment (MoCA)
- This is a brief tool developed to detect mild cognitive impairment that assesses a broader range of domains frequently affected in PD.
- It takes roughly 10–15 minutes to administer this cognitive screening tool.
- It is considered as a more sensitive screening instrument to detect early or mild cognitive impairment in PD compared to the MMSE.

3 Dementia Rating Scale
- This instrument is used to assess dementia in a wide range of neuropsychological conditions.

- It was originally developed to assess change in cognition in patients with dementia, but can be used to screen for dementia.
- The scale is divided into five subsections:
  - Attention
  - Initiation /perseveration
  - Construction
  - Conceptualization
  - Memory
- The scale takes about 20–30 minutes to complete and is most commonly used as a cognitive assessment prior to DBS surgery.

Sleep Assessment in PD

1. Epworth Sleep Scale
   - This is a validated self-report measure of daytime sleepiness covering any designated time period. It has been used in multiple disorders, including PD.
   - It assesses the likelihood of falling asleep in eight situations (e.g., sitting and reading, watching TV, talking to another person, riding as a passenger in a car).
   - Scoring on each item is 0 = would never doze; 1 = slight chance of dozing; 2 = moderate chance of dozing; 3 = high chance of dozing.
   - Since sleepiness is highly variable and may be normal, the scale assesses sleepiness severity, not pathology. A score >6 is considered indicative of sleepiness; >0 is very sleepy; >16 is dangerously sleepy.
2. Parkinson's Disease Sleep Scale (PDSS)

This scale uses a visual analogue score for each of 15 features commonly associated with sleep disturbance in PD:

- Overall quality of night's sleep (item 1)
- Sleep onset and maintenance insomnia (items 2 and 3)
- Nocturnal restlessness (items 4 and 5)
- Nocturnal psychosis (items 6 and 7)
- Nocturia (items 8 and 9)
- Nocturnal motor symptoms (items 10–13)
- Sleep refreshment (item 14)
- Daytime dozing (item 15)

Mood and Behavior

1 Geriatric Depression Scale
- The scale is a self-report measure designed to assess depressive symptoms in the elderly.
- The original version has 30 items. A short form (15 items) is also available, which correlates highly with the original.
- Items address affective and ideational features of depression, rather than somatic or vegetative features.
- A score <10 is within normal limits, scores of 10–19 indicate mild depressive symptoms, and scores of 20–30 suggest severe depressive symptoms.

2 Beck Depression Inventory (BDI)
- This is a self-rated scale used to measure the severity of depression.
- There are 21 items, evaluating key symptoms of depression.
  - Each item is followed by four statements, rated from 0 to 3. Patients are asked to circle the number by the statement that best describes their symptoms.
- The scores from each item are totaled, with a maximum score of 63.
- The BDI can be split into two subscales: cognitive-affective and somatic-performance.

3 Hamilton Depression Scale
- This is the most utilized rating scale for patients with primary depression.
- It consists of 21 items.
- Some items are rated on a 0–4 scale (0 = absent and 4 = most severe) while others are rated on a 0–2 scale (0 = absent or none and 2 = severe).
- The total score usually consists of the sum of the first 17 items because the last four items (diurnal variation, depersonalization and derealization, paranoid symptoms, and obsessive and compulsive symptoms) rarely occur in patients with depression.
- It usually takes 20–30 minutes to administer by a trained rater.

4 Parkinson Disease Fatigue Scale (PFS)
- This 16-item self-report instrument actually arose from statements by individuals with parkinsonism experiencing fatigue.

- The PFS was designed to survey the physical aspects of fatigue and their impact on the patient's daily function.
- The scale deliberately excludes emotional and cognitive features that may occur as part of the fatigue experience but which may also occur independently in parkinsonism.

5 Minnesota Impulsive Disorders Interview (MIDI), modified version

- This is a semistructured clinical interview assessing pathological gambling, compulsive buying, and compulsive sexual behavior.
- This has now become an important aspect in PD because of recent reports of impulse control behaviors as a side effect of anti-PD medications, especially the dopamine agonists.

6 Neuropsychiatric Inventory (NPI)

- The NPI evaluates behavioral abnormalities that occur in demented patients.
- It assesses behavior in 10 categories.
- Scoring is 0–3 in terms of severity and 0–4 for frequency. The severity and frequency scores for each category are then multiplied together and the scores for the categories are added to give a total score.
- An additional score is obtained for caregiver distress in each category.
- The assessment takes 15–30 minutes.

7 Brief Psychiatric Rating Scale

- This is a standardized scale used for the measurement of significant psychotic and nonpsychotic behavioral symptoms in patients with major mental disorders, mainly schizophrenia.
- There are different versions of the scale, but the 18-item scale is the most widely used. It assesses:
- Emotional states (anxiety, somatic concern, guilt, suspiciousness)
- Cognition (orientation, conceptual disorganization, and unusual thought content)
- Behavioral observations (emotional withdrawal, tension, mannerisms and posturing, grandiosity, depressive mood, hostility, hallucinations, motor retardation, uncooperativeness, blunted affect, excitement)
- Each item is scored on a 1–7 scale where 1 = not present and 7 = extremely severe.
- It takes 15–30 minutes given by a trained rater.

- While originally designed for schizophrenia patients, this is one of the most widely used scales in Parkinson trials concerning drugs for PD psychosis.

Patient Diaries

1 Patient diaries
  - The patient diary was developed as a tool to measure a person's motor state when the person is at home or is not being observed by a health care provider.
  - The diary is completed by the patient or sometimes the patient's caregiver.
  - One limitation of all self-administered diaries is that it is completely subjective. As well, patients with PD may be unaware of dyskinesias and, therefore, may not be able to provide an accurate assessment of their occurrence.
  - Training for diary completion by an experienced person is important.
  - Motor states assessed include:
    - Asleep
    - "Off"
    - "On"
    - "On" with nontroublesome dyskinesia
    - "On" with troublesome dyskinesia

SLEEP STUDIES

Sleep disturbance in Parkinson's disease is common and its cause can be multifactorial. Sleep studies are used to differentiate one cause from another. Individuals with PD may have difficulty falling and staying asleep, or staying awake. They may exhibit certain behaviors during sleep such as REM behavior disorder or periodic limb movement disorder.

Sleep studies are performed in a sleep laboratory that may be part of a hospital or may be a free-standing center. The lab includes a bedroom designed to simulate a comfortable, quiet, homelike sleeping environment. A trained sleep lab technician is the person who administers the tests.

Sleep studies include:

- Medical history and physical examination, which should be taken by the referring provider or sleep specialist before a study.

- Sleep diary, which should be completed by the patient for 2 weeks before a visit to a sleep laboratory.
- Polysomnogram study, which measures brain activity, eye movement, heart and respiratory rate and rhythm, body movements, oxygen and carbon dioxide levels, snoring, and the flow of air through the nose and mouth. Electrodes are placed on the head and body, a belt is worn to measure breathing patterns, and an oximeter is placed on the index finger to monitor blood oxygen levels. Polysomnogram recording equipment and video monitors record movements and activities while the patient sleeps.
- Multiple sleep latency test (MSLT), the gold standard in measuring stages of sleep in PD: This test is used to monitor when a person falls asleep and other behaviors through the night.
- Multiple wake test (MWT): This test monitors if a person can stay awake.

Study results are reviewed by a sleep specialist, often a neurologist or pulmonologist, and are usually available in 2 weeks.

Patient education includes avoiding caffeine, alcohol, and sedatives at minimum the day before a sleep study. Patients should be informed that glue will be used to attach electrodes to the body but that it will easily wash out. There is no pain associated with a sleep study.

SPEECH EVALUATION

A speech and language pathologist provides prevention, diagnosis, and rehabilitation of problems associated with speech, language, swallowing, and the cognitive aspects of communication. In Parkinson's disease individuals may experience problems with hypokinetic dysarthria (difficulty speaking clearly) and dysphagia (difficulty swallowing). In addition, mild cognitive changes can impact a person's linguistic ability.

Hypokinetic dysarthria occurs in over 50% of all individuals with PD at some point in their illness. It may be the presenting symptom of neurological disease in PD. Hypokinetic dysarthria is characterized by a breathy and hoarse voice and reduced loudness. Individuals with PD appear to have a perceptual disconnect between their actual loudness level and their own internal perception of loudness (they think they are speaking normally, or loudly, when they are actually quiet). Communication partners may have a hard time hearing their speech, especially at a distance, in a noisy environment, or on the telephone. Patients may also report avoiding social situations that require speech. The severity of speech disorders may not correspond to the duration of PD or severity of other motor symptoms. *Hyperkinetic dysarthria,* rather than *hypokinetic dysarthria,* may also be encountered. This most often occurs in the presence of dyskinesias, particularly after prolonged levodopa therapy.

Oropharyngeal dysphagia is reported in up to 95% of patients with PD, depending on the method of assessment. However, dysphagia is often unrecognized or underestimated by patients. Like dysarthria, the severity of dysphagia may not correspond to the duration of PD or severity of other motor symptoms. All stages of swallowing function can be affected in patients with PD including the oral, pharyngeal, and esophageal stages.

Areas of Assessment

- Phonation
- Resonance
- Voice pitch
- Articulation
- Linguistic ability
- Swallowing ability
- Hearing
- Facial expression

Treatment

Speech and Language

- Comprehensive voice evaluation
- Hearing assessment
- Lee Silverman Voice Treatment Program (LSVT), which has literature supporting its beneficial effects and is a popular treatment choice for individuals with PD and hypokinetic dysarthria
  - LSVT emphasizes phonatory effort and uses maximum performance tasks as the basis of intervention.
  - LSVT also recalibrates an individual's perceived level of effort with an emphasis on self-awareness.
  - LSVT is based upon the premise that treatment should be simple and intensive.

- Although intact cognition is a positive prognostic indicator of success, LSVT can also be beneficial for patients with cognitive deficits.
- Other treatments that may be appropriate, including rate control techniques and the use of delayed auditory feedback
- Augmentative-alternative communication (AAC) treatment approaches that may be beneficial particularly as dysarthria progresses
  - Voice amplifiers may be beneficial to increase vocal loudness.
  - Pacing boards may assist in rate control.
  - Alphabet boards may be an effective strategy to supplement speech and provide context for communication partners.
  - Other AAC strategies such as communication boards/notebooks, voice-output computer systems, and portable typing devices may also be used.

Swallowing

- Provide modified barium swallow evaluation.
- Provide strategies to improve swallowing techniques.
- Although dysphagia is common in PD, it rarely is severe enough to require an alternative means of nutritional support. However, gastrostomy may be considered for some patients as an efficient means to provide additional nutritional support. In some situations, oral intake may continue with the presence of a gastrostomy tube.

The Effect of Medications on Communication

- For most individuals with PD, pharmacological treatment does not appear to have a significant beneficial impact on speech production.
- Hyperkinetic dysarthria, often in the presence of dyskinesias after prolonged levodopa therapy, may also be encountered.

Surgical Treatments and Communication

- Surgical treatments for PD do not have consistent significant benefit for the communication impairments associated with PD.

Patient Educational Resources Prepared by Speech and Language Pathologists

Johnson, M. L. (2005). *Parkinson disease: Speech and swallowing* (2nd ed.). Miami, FL: National Parkinson Foundation.

Lee Silverman Voice Treatment (LSVT). Web site: www.lsvt.org

Ruddy, B. H., & Sapienza, C. (2003). *Speaking effectively: A strategic guide for speaking and swallowing.* New York: American Parkinson Disease Association.

Professional Organization for Speech and Language Pathologists

American Speech-Language-Hearing Association (ASHA)
2200 Research Blvd.
Rockville, MD 20850-3289
www.asha.org

SWALLOWING EVALUATION

Swallowing studies are ordered in individuals with dysphagia, particularly those at risk for aspiration pneumonia. Aspiration pneumonia can occur when food or liquid enters the airway rather than the esophagus during eating or drinking or sometimes with just excessive secretions. A speech and language pathologist (SLP) with experience in swallowing disorders will evaluate a person with dysphagia. Evaluation will include:

- History of disease process and symptoms
- Assessment of musculature involved in swallowing
- Observation of feeding patterns including rate of food intake, ability to chew, holding food or liquid in mouth, and ability to initiate a swallow

Two studies often performed include:

- Endoscopic assessment
- Modified barium swallow

An *endoscopic assessment* includes inserting a lighted scope through the nose, and viewing a swallow on a screen.

A *modified barium swallow* study utilizes X-rays and barium material to examine the function of the structures involved in swallowing. This test can help demonstrate anatomical or functional abnormalities with the mouth, pharynx, esophagus, and epiglottis. Barium is used due to its high density, which allows these structures to be visible on an X-ray.

Preparation for Testing

Usually no change in diet is necessary prior to testing. In the event that an upper gastrointestinal (GI) X-ray is to be performed, the patient should not eat after midnight on the day of the test. To lessen the risk of X-ray artifacts it is best to remove jewelry before the test.

Procedure

The procedure consists of having the patient swallow 16–20 ounces of a solution containing barium. An X-ray is performed in a variety of stages of swallowing. The entire examination may take around three hours including time spent discussing the results with the speech and language pathologist.

Results

The X-rays may help determine if there are changes in the mouth, pharynx, esophagus, or epiglottis. With PD, the rate and manner of swallowing can be affected. In the more advanced stages, aspiration of barium into the lungs may be documented on the study, suggesting that the individual is at an increased risk for aspiration pneumonia and probably should undergo dietary modifications. Less severe changes can be noted that will help guide eating habits as well. Aside from difficulties that occur with the progression of PD, differential diagnosis includes:

- Esophageal cancer
- Esophageal stricture
- Hiatal hernia (a portion of the stomach protrudes through the esophageal opening)
- Diverticulas (pouchlike sacs that protrude from the walls of an organ)
- Ulcers of the esophagus
- Achalasia (poor esophageal movement)

Special Considerations

- Constipation or worsening of constipation may occur following this study occasioned by the barium. If there is no bowel movement or/and barium doesn't pass through 2–3 days after the study, the participant should contact a physician.

UROLOGICAL TESTING IN PARKINSON'S DISEASE

Individuals who experience symptoms of an overactive bladder or other urinary problems related to Parkinson's disease will often be referred to a urologist for evaluation and testing. A complete urological workup may include the following:

Medical History

The medical history will include information on patterns of urination, history of illness, surgeries, pregnancies, and medication use. In Parkinson's disease careful attention is made to frequency and urgency of urination (including nocturia) as well as the use of medications with anticholinergic properties.

Physical Examination

The physical examination includes an assessment of the abdomen, rectum, genitals, and pelvis. Changes in reflexes and/or sensation are noted. Administration of a *cough stress test* differentiates stress incontinence from urge incontinence.

Urinalysis

Urinalysis is done to identify an infection or other problem.

Urodynamic Testing

A cystometer is used to measure the anatomic and functional status of the bladder and urethra. Cystometry measures bladder pressure and capacity.

Postvoid Residual

Catheterization is used to measure the amount of urine that remains in the bladder after voiding. The patient is asked to void and then a postvoid residual (PVR) is measured. Repeated PVR measures of greater than 100 mL suggest inadequate bladder emptying.

Uroflowmetry

This test measures the pattern of urine flow.

Endoscopic Testing

A cystoscopy may be performed to survey the inside of the bladder to be certain that bladder lesions or foreign bodies are not present. This would only be done if symptoms suggested these problems.

After a thorough evaluation, recommendations for treatment are made by the urologist in consultation with the neurologist.

SECTION III

Treatment

A Pharmacological Management

GOALS OF THERAPY

The primary objective of medical management is to maximize control over the target signs and symptoms of PD. This is accomplished by first selecting the appropriate drug(s) for each symptom and then adjusting the dose and frequency of drug administration over time. Parkinson's symptoms as well as response to medication are highly variable from person to person requiring an individualized approach.

The patient's therapeutic response to any individual drug may change over time and requires regular visits and frequent communication between the medical team, the patient, and caregiver(s) to maintain the best management of the disease with the fewest side effects possible. All health care professionals regardless of prescription authority can play a role in medication management. This is particularly important for health care providers who observe patients over longer periods of time, such as a nurse who is caring for a person in an assisted living facility or a physical therapist during a treatment session.

Health care professionals are prepared to:

- Assess and monitor signs and symptoms over a period of time
- Evaluate responses to treatment

- Provide accurate information to the prescriber
- Facilitate communication between patient/family and multiple health care disciplines
- Provide patient/family (and coworker) education
- Assess patient/family coping strategies, define unmet needs, and provide support in accessing resources

Patients and families require extensive education and support to properly manage medications. Medications, usually more than one, are administered at frequent intervals during the day. Schedules can be complex. Side effects are often difficult to differentiate from signs and symptoms. In general the following recommendations should be shared with patients and families:

- Keep an accurate and updated list of all medications. Include medications previously used including name, dose, how long it was taken, and reason for discontinuation.
- Understand the action, dosing schedule, and side-effect profile of each medication.
- Understand how to differentiate PD symptoms from adverse effects of treatment.
- Know when to contact a health care provider.
- Utilize diaries to record motor state over a 24-hour period. These tools can empower the patient and family in describing the response to medications and communicating complaints clearly and factually.

SPECIAL CONSIDERATIONS FOR HEALTH CARE PROFESSIONALS

- Medications must be administered on time.
- Careful consideration must be made as to the timing of doses and activities of daily living.
- Observation and documentation must be made of doses' desired effect, lack of effect, and/or presence of side effects.
  - How long does it take before medication kicks in?
  - How long does each dose last?
  - Is wearing off gradual or abrupt, predictable or unpredictable?

- How do the fluctuations affect the individual from a functional and psychological standpoint?
- The difference between "on" and "off" must be understood.
- Differentiation must be made between tremor (a PD symptom) and dyskinesia (a medication side effect).
- Note must be made that stress, sleep deprivation, infection, dehydration, and changes in coexisting diseases can affect an individual's response to medications.

AGENTS USED FOR MOTOR CONTROL

Amantadine (SYMMETREL®)

Amantadine is an antiviral medication that has been used to prevent illnesses such as influenza type A, and has also found a place in the treatment of Parkinson's disease. It is used to alleviate mild symptoms of PD including tremor and rigidity and most often to treat dyskinesia, involuntary movements associated with too much dopamine in the brain.

The exact mechanism is not well understood. Amantadine increases dopaminergic activity in the peripheral and central nervous system by augmenting the release and inhibiting the cellular reuptake of dopamine. Its antidyskinetic effect has been attributed to its possible antiglutamate mechanism of action.

Targets of therapy of amantadine include:

- Mild improvement of Parkinson's symptoms when beginning the medication
- Reduction of dyskinesia

Side Effects

As with most medications, side effects may occur when treatment starts, when the dose is changed, or at any time; not everyone will experience side effects. Potential side effects include:

- Difficulty concentrating
- Dizziness or lightheadedness
- Headache
- Confusion

Table 3.1

AMANTADINE (SYMMETREL®)
Available as: Capsules 100 mg, liquid syrup 50 mg/5 ml liquid
Dosing issues: Initiate dose 100 mg bid increase up to 100 mg tid

- Loss of appetite
- Nausea
- Livedo reticularis (purplish red, netlike, blotchy spots on skin often on legs)
- Edema
- Constipation
- Diarrhea
- Insomnia
- Blurred vision
- Hallucinations

Special Considerations

- Amantadine should be used cautiously in patients with cardiac and renal disease (see Table 3.1).

Please refer to drug reference guides for dose ranges and a complete list of drug interactions and adverse effects.

Apomorphine (APOKYN®)

Apomorphine is a non-ergot dopamine agonist used in the treatment of acute disabling "off" periods. It is administered by subcutaneous injection by the patient or a caregiver. The drug works rapidly with relief of parkinsonian symptoms, typically within 10–20 minutes. Apomorphine must be taken, at least initially, with the antiemetic medication trimethobenzamide hydrochloride (Tigan®) or domperidone (Motilium®, if available) to prevent nausea and vomiting. Trimethobenzamide 300-mg tablets should be taken 3 times daily for 3 days prior to the first dose of apomorphine and should continue for at least two months when apomorphine is being used.

Initial administration and dose titration is done under the careful supervision of a physician. The protocol is described at the end of this module. Apomorphine can be administered up to 5 times a day. Doses greater than 6 mg are not recommended (see Table 3.2).

Targets of therapy of apomorphine include:

- End-of-dose wearing-off episodes
- Unpredictable "off" episodes
- Painful "off" periods

Side Effects

As with most medications, side effects may occur when treatment starts, when the dose is changed, or at any time; not everyone will experience side effects. Potential side effects include:

- Nausea
- Vomiting
- Dizziness
- Postural hypotension
- Somnolence
- Yawning
- Injection site reactions
- Dyskinesia
- Hallucinations
- Falls

Special Considerations

- Apomorphine should not be used in patients allergic to sulfites.
- It should not be used in patients receiving serotonin antagonists (e.g., ondansetron, granisetron, dolasetron, palonosetron, and alosetron).
- A comprehensive support program (Apokyn Circle of Care™) is available to health care professionals to provide education and support to patients and health care professionals (www.apokyn.com).
- Apokyn is useful in patients who are temporarily unable to swallow to take their oral PD medications, for example, NPO for surgery (see Table 3.3).

Table 3.2

APOMORPHINE (APOKYN®) TITRATION DONE UNDER MEDICAL SUPERVISION

FIRST TEST DOSE 0.2 mL	IF 1st DOSE IS INEFFECTIVE TRY 2nd TEST DOSE OF 0.4mL AT NEXT OBSERVED "OFF" PERIOD	IF 0.4 mL DOSE IS NOT TOLERATED TRY 0.3mL DOSE AT ANOTHER "OFF" PERIOD
Ascertain that the patient is in the "off" condition. ↓ Obtain blood pressure (BP) in supine and standing positions prior to dosing. Patient or caregiver administers 0.2 mL test dose. ↓ Obtain BP in supine and standing positions at 20, 40, and 60 minutes following dosing. If the test dose is tolerated, and response is noted, the starting dose should be 0.2 mL, to be used as needed. ↓ As needed, this starting dose can be titrated upward at increments of 0.1 mL every few days. This can be done on an outpatient basis. ↓ Those who develop clinically significant orthostatic hypotension with 0.2 mL test dose should not be considered candidates for treatment with Apokyn (apomorphine).	This dose is administered to the patient who tolerates the 0.2 mL test dose, however, does not demonstrate a response. ↓ Do not administer sooner than 2 hours following initial 0.2 mL test dose. Obtain BP in supine and standing positions prior to dosing. Patient or caregiver administers 0.4 mL test dose. ↓ Obtain BP in supine and standing positions at 20, 40, and 60 minutes following dosing. ↓ If the 0.4 mL test dose is tolerated, regardless of whether or not there is a response, the starting dose should be 0.3 mL, used as needed. ↓ If needed, this dose can be increased in increments of 0.1 mL every few days. This can be done on an outpatient basis. Efficacy and tolerability will need to be assessed from time to time.	Dose of 0.3 mL should be administered to those who do not tolerate the 0.4 mL test dose. ↓ Do not administer sooner than 2 hours following the 0.4 mL test dose. Obtain BP in supine and standing positions prior to dosing. Patient or caregiver administers the 0.3 mL test dose. ↓ Obtain BP in supine and standing positions at 20, 40, and 60 minutes following dosing. ↓ If the 0.3 mL test dose is tolerated, the starting dose should be 0.2 mL, used as needed. ↓ If needed, after a few days this dose can be increased to 0.3 mL. This can be done on an outpatient basis. Assess efficacy and tolerability from time to time. The dose in these patients generally should not be increased to 0.4 mL on an outpatient basis.

Table 3.3

APOMORPHINE (APOKYN®)
Injectable formulation 10 mg/mL, available in a pen-type injector (SC = under the skin)
Primarily used to treat acute "off" periods. Requires specific/detailed training.
Contra-indicated in patients allergic to sulfites or if treated with 5HT3 antagonists such as ondansetron, granisetron, etc.

Please refer to drug reference guides for dose ranges and a complete list of drug interactions and adverse effects.

Benztropine (COGENTIN®)

Benztropine is an anticholinergic drug used in PD primarily to treat tremor early in the disease or tremor that does not adequately respond to other anti-Parkinson medication. This medication works by blocking the brain chemical acetylcholine and creating a *balance* with dopamine. It, along with the other anticholinergic therapies, has side effects including urinary retention, blurred vision, confusion, dry mouth, and constipation. Elderly populations are particularly susceptible to anticholinergic side effects. A careful assessment of the patient's risk-to-benefit ratio should be performed before initiating treatment with anticholinergic drugs.

Targets of therapy of benztropine include:

- Tremor
- Dystonia
- Rigidity

Side Effects

As with most medications, side effects may occur when treatment starts, when the dose is changed, or at any time; not everyone will experience side effects. Potential side effects include:

- Blurred vision
- Urinary retention

Table 3.4

BENZTROPINE MESYLATE (COGENTIN®)
How supplied: Tablets 0.5 mg, 1.0 mg, 2.0 mg

- Confusion
- Memory loss
- Listlessness
- Sedation
- Decreased appetite
- Dry mouth
- Nausea
- Vomiting
- Diarrhea
- Constipation
- Increased eye sensitivity to light
- Dry eyes
- Weight loss
- Hallucination

Special Considerations

- When dosing these agents, start low and go slow. A slow upward titration is done until tremor and/or dystonia improves or until side effects develop (see Table 3.4).
- This medication should not be stopped suddenly but should be tapered.
- This medication should not be prescribed in individuals with glaucoma.

Please refer to drug reference guides for dose ranges and a complete list of drug interactions and adverse effects.

Bromocriptine (PARLODEL®)

Bromocriptine is as an ergot-derived dopamine agonist that mimics the effect of dopamine by stimulating dopamine receptors directly. The first dopamine agonist was used to treat PD symptoms; it is rarely used now because of its cost, potential ergot effect, and availability of newer dopamine agonists.

In early Parkinson's disease it provides sufficient relief of symptoms delaying the need to introduce carbidopa/levodopa. In moderate to advanced Parkinson's disease it is used in combination with carbidopa/levodopa.

Targets of therapy of bromocriptine include:

- Rigidity
- Bradykinesia
- Tremor

Side Effects

As with most medications, side effects may occur when treatment starts, when the dose is changed, or at any time; not everyone will experience side effects. Potential side effects include:

- Orthostatic hypotension
- Dizziness
- Nausea
- Headache
- Edema often of feet and ankles
- Fatigue
- Confusion
- Hallucinations
- Compulsive disorders
- Dyskinesia
- Ergotism
- Somnolence

Special Considerations

- Dose titration is done slowly to decrease the risk of postural hypotension.
- It may take 2–4 weeks to notice symptom relief (see Table 3.5).

Please refer to drug reference guides for dose ranges and a complete list of drug interactions and adverse effects.

Table 3.5

BROMOCRIPTINE MESYLATE (PARLODEL®)
Available as: 2.5 mg tablet or 5 mg capsule

Carbidopa/Levodopa (SINEMET®, SINEMET CR®, PARCOPA®)

The primary drug used to relieve Parkinson symptoms is a combination of carbidopa and levodopa. It is clearly the most efficacious pharmacologic treatment for PD to date. In the brain, levodopa is converted to dopamine, a neurotransmitter that is deficient in Parkinson's disease. Carbidopa allows levodopa to enter the brain with fewer side effects such as nausea, vomiting, and decreased blood pressure. The dose is written as a fraction with the top number representing the amount of carbidopa and the bottom number representing the amount of levodopa.

The initial use and dosage of carbidopa/levodopa is debated in the medical community. The decision to initiate therapy depends on a person's age, the extent to which the person's symptoms affect mobility, ability to perform activities of daily living, mood, cognition, and employment. Delay of therapy with levodopa *potentially* delays the onset of motor fluctuations including wearing off, dyskinesia, and "on-off." Younger patients (typically less than 60 years old) are slightly more prone to developing these motor fluctuations than older PD patients. However, regardless of age, individuals should receive treatment with carbidopa/levodopa when PD symptoms affect quality of life and functional status, especially when other PD medications do not provide significant benefit.

Targets of therapy of carbidopa/levodopa include:

- Rigidity (muscle stiffness)
- Tremor—levodopa may not eliminate tremor completely
- Bradykinesia (slowness of moving)
- Gait disturbance (slowed walking, leg dragging)
- Hypomimia (reduced facial expression)
- Micrographia (small handwriting)

Carbidopa/levodopa does not treat:

- Postural instability (poor balance)
- Hypophonia (soft voice)
- Sexual dysfunction
- Excessive sweating
- Seborrhea (oily skin)
- Constipation
- Dementia

Side Effects

As with most medications, side effects may occur when treatment starts, when the dose is changed, or at any time; not everyone will experience side effects. Potential side effects include:

- Nausea
- Vomiting
- Postural hypotension
- Dyskinesias (abnormal involuntary dancelike or twisting movements)
- Confusion
- Hallucinations
- Dystonia (abnormal twisting posturing of certain body parts)
- Wearing-off effect
- "On-off" effect
- Somnolence
- Insomnia
- Skin rash (which may be related to tablet dye color, typically the yellow dye when it occurs)
- Dry mouth
- Repetitive or compulsive behaviors (such as doing an activity/hobby over and over)
- Increased desire to medicate with more carbidopa/levodopa

Long-term side effects may include:

- A wearing-off effect: when symptoms return before the next scheduled dose. To manage this side effect the doctor may increase the dose/frequency or add an additional agent.

- Dyskinesia: This is a term used to describe abnormal movements in the neck, trunk of the body, and upper extremities. Usually a reduction or redistribution of doses must be made.
- "On-Off" phenomenon: "On" periods are when movements are as normal as possible for the individual. Dyskinesias may be present during "on" periods. "Off" periods are when Parkinson symptoms have returned (bradykinesia, rigidity, and tremor).

Special Considerations

- High-protein meals decrease the absorption of carbidopa/levodopa, and the medication is most effective on an empty stomach. However, taking it on an empty stomach may increase the risk of nausea. If the nausea is intolerable this medication may be taken with a nonprotein snack, such as crackers or fruit.
- Carbidopa/levodopa should be used with caution in patients with a history of melanoma.
- Always take this medication with a full glass of water or juice (not necessary with Parcopa).
- Never abruptly stop carbidopa/levodopa without consulting a health care provider (risk of malignant hyperthermia).
- Since carbidopa/levodopa is taken at frequent intervals during the day, patients often use special wristwatches or pillboxes with multiple alarm settings (see Table 3.6).

Table 3.6

CARBIDOPA/LEVODOPA (SINEMET®)

Available as: 10/100, 25/100, 25/250
Dosing issues: Tablet is scored
Take 1/2 hour to 1 hour before meals or 2 hours after meals
Take with a full glass of water or juice

Sinemet CR® Controlled-release or long-acting form
Available as: 25/100, 50/200
Dosing issues: Never chew, crush, or cut the controlled-release/long-acting form (CR)
Take with a full glass of water or juice

Parcopa® orally disintegrating tablet that dissolves on the tongue
Available as: 10/100, 25/100, 25/250
Dosing issues: Can be taken with/without fluid or drink

Please refer to drug reference guides for dose ranges and a complete list of drug interactions and adverse effects.

Entacapone (COMTAN®, STALEVO®)

Entacapone is a catechol-O-methyl transferase (COMT) inhibitor, a medication that works by blocking COMT, an enzyme that breaks down dopamine, thereby increasing dopamine availability. In order for the medication to work, entacapone must be used in combination with carbidopa/levodopa. A tablet containing both carbidopa/levodopa and entacapone exists as Stalevo®.

Targets of therapy of entacapone include:

- Wearing off or "off" periods associated with long-term management of carbidopa/levodopa and disease progression.
- It remains under investigation whether adding entacapone prior to experiencing wearing off is beneficial.

Side Effects

As with most medications, side effects may occur when treatment starts, when the dose is changed, or at any time; not everyone will experience side effects. Potential side effects include:

- Diarrhea
- Discoloration of urine (dark orange color)
- Discoloration of teeth and nails
- Dyskinesia
- Nausea
- Hallucinations
- Confusion
- Orthostatic hypotension

Special Considerations

- Diarrhea if associated with entacapone typically appears 6–8 weeks after the initiation of treatment. The nature of this side effect often leads to discontinuation of the drug.
- Patients and families should be informed of discoloration of urine as well as orange staining of the teeth or nails that may occur from the tablets. It is best to avoid chewing, crushing, or splitting the tablets.

Table 3.7

ENTACAPONE (COMTAN®)
How supplied: 200 mg tablets. Take one tablet with each dose of carbidopa/levodopa up to 8 doses.
Carbidopa/levodopa/entacapone (Stalevo®) Tablets containing: # mg carbidopa/# mg levodopa/# mg entacapone
Available Doses: Stalevo 50: 12.5 mg/50 mg/200 mg Stalevo 100: 25 mg/100 mg/200 mg Stalevo 150: 37.5 mg/150 mg/200 mg Stalevo 200: 50 mg/200 mg/200 mg

- Should be used with caution in individuals with elevated liver enzymes or hepatic disease (see Table 3.7).

Please refer to drug reference guides for dose ranges and a complete list of drug interactions and adverse effects.

Pramipexole (MIRAPEX®)

Pramipexole is a non-ergot dopamine agonist that mimics the effect of dopamine by stimulating dopamine receptors (specifically D2 and D3 receptors). It is approved for early and advanced PD and can be used by itself or with other anti-Parkinson medications such as carbidopa/levodopa.

Targets of therapy of pramipexole include:

- Rigidity
- Bradykinesia
- Tremor

Side Effects

As with most medications, side effects may occur when treatment starts, when the dose is changed, or at any time; not everyone will experience side effects. Potential side effects include:

- Postural hypotension
- Dizziness
- Nausea

Table 3.8

PRAMIPEXOLE DIHYDROCHLORIDE (MIRAPEX®)
Available as: 0.125 mg, 0.25 mg, 0.5 mg, 1.0 mg, 1.5 mg tablets

- Vomiting
- Somnolence
- Sudden sleep attacks
- Insomnia
- Confusion
- Hallucinations
- Compulsive disorders
- Constipation
- Edema

Special Considerations

- Sudden-onset sleep. Falling asleep while eating, having a conversation, or in the middle of another activity have been reported; as a result there is an increased risk of accident if driving or operating machinery. Patients should be informed of this risk at initiation of therapy, particularly how it relates to driving.
- Impulse control behaviors including gambling, hypersexuality, and buying disorders have emerged or increased with the use of pramipexole as well as other dopaminergic agents. A complete assessment of these behaviors should be done at the initiation and during the course of treatment.
- Dose titration is done slowly with a starting dose of 0.125 mg three times a day, gradually increasing by 0.125 mg/dose every 5–7 days. Dose range is 1.5–4.5 mg/day with a maximum daily dose of 6 mg (see Table 3.8).

Please refer to drug reference guides for dose ranges and a complete list of drug interactions and adverse effects.

Propranolol (INDERAL®)

Normally used to treat high blood pressure, beta blockers such as propranolol may decrease some types of tremor (see Table 3.9). Propranolol

Table 3.9

PROPRANOLOL (INDERAL®)	
Available as:	Inderal 10 mg, 20 mg, 40 mg, 80 mg and 120 mg tablets Inderal-LA 60 mg, 80 mg, 120 mg, 160 mg tablets Propranolol 10 mg, 20 mg, 40 mg, 80 mg tablets

is more effective in treating *action* or *postural* tremor than the more typical *resting* tremor in Parkinson's disease. Some individuals with PD have both action and resting tremor. Propranolol may benefit these individuals. When used daily it is possible to use a longer-acting, once-a-day formulation. The more immediate formulation is taken once, twice, three, or four times a day, but its effects only last a few hours. Propranolol can be taken as needed at a very low dose to help in stressful situations that may aggravate tremor such as eating out in restaurants, public speaking, or even visiting a health care provider.

Targets of therapy of propranolol include:

- Hypertension
- Tremor

Side Effects

As with most medications, side effects may occur when treatment starts, when the dose is changed, or at any time; not everyone will experience side effects. Potential side effects include:

- Dizziness or light-headedness due to a reduced heart rate and/or a drop in blood pressure; close monitoring of the pulse (typically avoid dropping the pulse less than 60 beats per minute) and blood pressure is needed, often necessitating a home blood pressure kit with involvement by a primary care physician
- Difficulty sleeping
- Excessive tiredness
- Nausea
- Vomiting
- Rash
- Diarrhea

- Constipation
- Depression

Special Considerations

- The primary care physician familiar with the patient's cardiac status may be consulted before the use of propranolol

Please refer to drug reference guides for dose ranges and a complete list of drug interactions and adverse effects.

Rasagiline (AZILECT®)

Rasagiline is a monoamine oxidase (MAO) type-B inhibitor that decreases the metabolism or breakdown of dopamine. This agent is used alone to treat mild early PD symptoms or in combination with levodopa later in the disease. This agent has also been studied for its potential to slow disease progression in PD. The official results are still unavailable at the time of this writing.

Targets of therapy of rasagiline include:

- Rigidity
- Tremor
- Bradykinesia

Side Effects

As with most medications, side effects may occur when treatment starts, when the dose is changed, or at any time; not everyone will experience side effects. Potential side effects include:

- Gastrointestinal upset
- Increase in dopaminergic symptoms including dyskinesia, dystonia, and hallucinations when used with carbidopa/levodopa
- Confusion

Special Considerations

- Rasagiline should not be taken with meperidine (Demerol®). Patients scheduled for elective surgery or a procedure, such as colonoscopy, should discuss this medication with their health care providers.

Table 3.10

RASAGILINE (AZILECT®)
Available as: 0.5 mg and 1.0 mg tablets

- Use cautiously with SSRIs due to increased risk of confusion.
- Avoid cough, cold, and allergy medications containing dextromethorphan (DM) or pseudoephedrine.
- Omeprazole and ciprofloxacin may alter the potency of this medication.
- The U.S. Food and Drug Administration cautions the intake of tyramine-rich foods including aged meats, soybean products, aged cheeses, and tap beer with rasagiline due to a potential interaction. However, clinical trials with "tyramine challenge" have not shown any significant adverse effects when rasagiline is mixed with tyramine (see Table 3.10).

Please refer to drug reference guides for dose ranges and a complete list of drug interactions and adverse effects.

Ropinirole (REQUIP®, REQUIP XL®)

Ropinirole is a non-ergot dopamine agonist that mimics the effect of dopamine by stimulating dopamine receptors. It is approved for early and advanced PD and can be used alone or with other anti-Parkinson medications such as carbidopa/levodopa.

Targets of therapy of ropinirole include:

- Rigidity
- Bradykinesia
- Tremor
- Restless legs syndrome

Side Effects

As with most medications, side effects may occur when treatment starts, when the dose is changed, or at any time; not everyone will experience side effects. Potential side effects include:

- Nausea
- Vomiting
- Somnolence (including "sleep attacks")
- Impulse control disorders (such as excessive gambling, spending, eating, or sex)
- Dizziness
- Confusion
- Orthostatic hypotension
- Dyskinesia
- Drowsiness
- Headache
- Hallucinations or paranoid behavior
- Weight gain or leg swelling

Special Considerations

- The dosing titration schedule of ropinirole is implemented slowly to avoid side effects. Therapeutic effect may take several weeks. Patients and family members should be informed of this.
- Sudden-onset sleep: falling asleep while eating, having a conversation, or in the middle of another activity have been reported; as a result there is an increase risk of accident if driving or operating machinery. Patients should be informed of this risk at initiation of therapy, particularly how it relates to driving.
- Impulse control behaviors including gambling, hypersexuality, and buying disorders have emerged or increased with the use of dopaminergic agents. A complete assessment of these behaviors should be done at the initiation of and during the course of treatment (see Table 3.11).

Please refer to drug reference guides for dose ranges and a complete list of drug interactions and adverse effects.

Table 3.11

ROPINIROLE (REQUIP®, REQUIP XL®)
Available as: 0.25 mg, 0.5 mg, 1, 2, 3, 4, and 5 mg; or as 2 mg, 4 mg, 8 mg in the XL extended-release formulation

Rotigotine (NEUPRO®)

Rotigotine was an approved dopamine agonist used to treat the motor symptoms of PD. However, it was recently pulled from the market by the FDA due to irregularity in drug delivery that resulted as part of the manufacturing process. As of this writing, return to the market is expected shortly. Dopamine agonists mimic the effect of dopamine by stimulating receptors directly. It is the first transdermal patch used in PD treatment. A major advantage of this dopamine agonist is the once-daily application. This is an important quality-of-life issue for individuals who take medications several times a day. In the United States, it is approved for use as a first agent in early PD. In Europe, it is also approved as an adjunctive medication in moderate to advanced PD.

Target of therapy of rotigotine includes:

- Rigidity
- Bradykinesia
- Tremor

Side Effects

As with most medications, side effects may occur when treatment starts, when the dose is changed, or at any time; not everyone will experience side effects. Potential side effects include:

- Postural hypotension
- Skin reactions at patch site
- Nausea
- Vomiting
- Hallucinations and paranoia
- Somnolence (including sleep attacks)
- Weight gain

Special Considerations

- The transdermal patch is applied every 24 hours.
- The application site should be rotated, ideally not using the same site within 14 days.
- The transdermal patch should not be exposed to natural sunlight.

Table 3.12

ROTIGOTINE (NEUPRO®) TRANSDERMAL PATCH
Available as: 2 mg, 4 mg, 6 mg patch; presently off the market

- Vigilance for idiosyncratic side effects seen in dopamine agonists should also be applied when using the rotigotine patch, such as sleep attacks, weight gain, and impulse control disorders (like excessive spending, gambling, sex, or eating). (See Table 3.12.)

Please refer to drug reference guides for dose ranges and a complete list of drug interactions and adverse effects.

Selegiline (ELDEPRYL®, DEPRENYL®, ZELAPAR®)

Selegiline is an MAO type-B inhibitor that decreases the metabolism or breakdown of dopamine, making it last longer in the brain. This agent is used alone to treat mild, early PD symptoms or in combination with levodopa later in the disease. In 2006 Zelapar®, an orally disintegrating selegiline tablet, was approved. This new formulation is dissolved quickly in the saliva and is absorbed directly through the oral mucosa.

Targets of therapy of selegiline include:

- Rigidity
- Bradykinesia
- Tremor

Side Effects

As with most medications, side effects may occur when treatment starts, when the dose is changed, or at any time; not everyone will experience side effects. Potential side effects include:

- Insomnia
- Gastrointestinal upset
- Increase in dopaminergic symptoms including dyskinesia, dystonia, and hallucinations when used with carbidopa/levodopa
- Confusion

Table 3.13

SELEGILINE	
Selegiline (Eldepryl®)	**Orally-disintegrating selegiline (Zelapar®)**
Available as: 5 mg tablets	Available as: 1.25 mg tablets
	Special Consideration: Instruct the patient to let the medication absorb under the tongue. Patient should not eat or drink anything for 5 minutes after medication intake to fully absorb the medication

Special Considerations

- Selegiline should not be taken with meperidine (Demerol®). Patients scheduled for elective surgery or a procedure such as colonoscopy should discuss this medication with their health care providers.
- Use cautiously with SSRIs due to increased risk of confusion.
- Last dose of selegiline should not be taken after 2:00 P.M. due to an increased risk of insomnia (see Table 3.13).

Please refer to drug reference guides for dose ranges and a complete list of drug interactions and adverse effects.

Tolcapone (TASMAR®)

Tolcapone is a COMT inhibitor, a medication that works by blocking catechol-O-methyltransferase, an enzyme that breaks down levodopa in the gut, thereby increasing its availability for absorption. This action increases the amount of levodopa that reaches the brain for conversion to dopamine. In order for tolcapone to work, it must be used in combination with carbidopa/levodopa. This agent was previously removed by the FDA due to rare cases of hepatic necrosis. It is now FDA-approved with guidelines for careful monitoring of liver enzymes.

Targets of therapy of tolcapone include:

- Wearing off or "off" periods associated with long-term management of carbidopa/levodopa and disease progression.

Side Effects

As with most medications, side effects may occur when treatment starts, when the dose is changed, or at any time; not everyone will experience side effects. Potential side effects include:

- Nausea
- Dyskinesia
- Excessive dreaming
- Diarrhea
- Orthostatic hypotension
- Vomiting
- Increased sweating
- Liver function abnormalities
- Urine discoloration
- Hallucinations
- Sleep disturbance

Special Considerations

- The FDA has established liver function monitoring guidelines. Blood test monitoring of liver enzymes should be performed before initiating tolcapone and at periodic intervals as described below.
- Tolcapone should be used as an adjunct only in PD patients on carbidopa/levodopa who are experiencing symptom fluctuation and who are not responding to or are not appropriate candidates for other therapies.

Tolcapone Liver Monitoring Guidelines

- Tolcapone administration requires baseline serum glutamic-pyruvic transaminase (SGPT/ALT) and serum glutamic-oxaloacetic transaminase (SGOT/AST), with levels checked every month for 6 months and as needed thereafter.
- If the dose is increased to 200 mg 3 times per day, liver enzyme monitoring should take place before increasing the dose.
- Because of the rare possibility of acute fulminant hepatitis with tolcapone, it should not be initiated if the patient exhibits clinical evidence of liver disease or 2 SGPT/ALT or SGOT/ALT values greater than the upper limit of normal.

Table 3.14

TOLCAPONE (TASMAR®)
Available doses: Tablet, 100 mg, 200 mg

- Tolcapone should be discontinued if the ALT or AST levels exceed the upper limit of normal or if clinical signs or symptoms suggest the onset of hepatic failure (persistent nausea, fatigue, lethargy, anorexia, jaundice, dark urine, pruritus, and right upper quadrant tenderness). (See Table 3.14.)

Please refer to drug reference guides for dose ranges and a complete list of drug interactions and adverse effects.

Trihexyphenidyl (ARTANE®)

Trihexyphenidyl is an anticholinergic drug used in PD primarily to treat tremor early in the disease or tremor that does not adequately respond to other anti-Parkinson medication. This medication works by blocking the brain chemical acetylcholine and creating a balance with the dopamine. It along with the other anticholinergic therapies has side effects including urinary retention, blurred vision, confusion, and constipation. Elderly populations are particularly susceptible. A careful risk-to-benefit ratio should be performed before initiating treatment.

Targets of therapy of trihexyphenidyl include:

- Tremor
- Dystonia
- Rigidity

Side Effects

As with most medications, side effects may occur when treatment starts, when the dose is changed, or at any time; not everyone will experience side effects. Potential side effects include:

- Blurred vision
- Urinary retention
- Confusion

Table 3.15

TRIHEXYPHENIDYL (ARTANE®)
How supplied: 2 mg and 5 mg tablets, Liquid 2 mg/5 ml

- Listlessness
- Sedation
- Decreased appetite
- Dry mouth
- Nausea
- Vomiting
- Diarrhea
- Constipation
- Increased eye sensitivity to light
- Dry eyes
- Weight Loss

Special Considerations

- When dosing these agents, start low and go slow. Three times daily dosing is the target regimen; however, twice daily dosing may be useful if the patient is having difficulty tolerating the medication. A slow upward titration is done until tremor and/or dystonia improves or until side effects develop.
- This medication should not be stopped suddenly but should be tapered.
- This medication should not be prescribed in individuals with glaucoma (see Table 3.15).

Please refer to drug reference guides for dose ranges and a complete list of drug interactions and adverse effects.

AGENTS USED FOR DEPRESSION: SELECTIVE SEROTONIN REUPTAKE INHIBITORS

There are three neurotransmitters that have been implicated in the pathogenesis of depression. These include serotonin, dopamine, and norepinephrine. When these neurotransmitters become unbalanced, for instance, if the supply of serotonin is low, then symptoms may occur in a patient such as sadness, guilt, changes in sleeping and/or eating patterns, decreased energy, decreased concentration, and loss of pleasure in activities that may have once been pleasurable. A class of agents known as selective serotonin reuptake inhibitors, or SSRIs, was developed in order to help correct the potential imbalances of these neurotransmitters with serotonin in particular because it is thought to be the primary mediator that underlies mood.

The SSRIs represent an important class of newer antidepressants. SSRIs work by allowing the body to make the best use of the reduced amounts of serotonin that it has at the time. There are currently six agents that fall into this category, and research indicates that they each have varying minor effects on other neurotransmitters as well, mainly norepinephrine and dopamine.

SSRIs are often the best choice for a depressed person with PD who also has cognitive difficulties and experiences excessive daytime sleepiness. These drugs are thought to have an "alerting effect," and may counteract the sedative component of traditional anti-Parkinson medications.

The antidepressant effects of SSRIs take several weeks to occur, and some patients may not experience the full benefit until after 8 weeks have lapsed. However, symptoms of depression may begin to improve within the first several days. For instance, in the first week of starting an SSRI, patients report that sleeping and eating patterns improve. During the following several days patients may find themselves with more energy. Improvements in mood and mentality may occur after 3 weeks with the full benefit expected after 4–6 weeks.

SSRIs available include:

- Fluoxetine (Prozac®)
- Sertraline (Zoloft ®)
- Paroxetine (Paxil®)
- Fluvoxamine (Luvox®)
- Citalopram (Celexa®)
- Escitalopram (Lexapro®)

Fluvoxamine (Luvox®) is an SSRI that is not readily prescribed, because it is associated with more side effects and drug interactions than the other five. A patient with Parkinson's disease typically needs to be on numerous medications; therefore, side effects and drug interactions should be minimized. Fluoxetine (Prozac®) may increase Parkinson symptoms more than other available SSRIs. Therefore, only the other four antidepressants will be discussed in this section: sertraline (Zoloft®), paroxetine (Paxil®), citalopram (Celexa®), and escitalopram (Lexapro®). See Table 3.26 for side-effect information on antidepressants for PD.

Sertraline (ZOLOFT®)

Sertraline is an antidepressant classified as an SSRI (see Table 3.16).

Targets of therapy of sertraline include:

- Depression
- Posttraumatic stress disorder
- Obsessive-compulsive disorder
- Panic disorder
- Premenstrual dysphoric disorder
- Social anxiety disorder

Side Effects

As with most medications, side effects may occur when treatment starts, when the dose is changed, or at any time; not everyone will experience side effects. Potential side effects include:

- Diarrhea
- Dry mouth
- Nausea
- Blurred vision
- Vomiting
- Gas or bloating

Table 3.16

SERTRALINE (ZOLOFT®)
Available as: 25 mg, 50 mg, 100 mg tablets 20 mg/mL oral concentrate (12% alcohol)
Oral concentrate: Must mix with 4 oz of water, ginger ale, lemon/lime soda, lemonade, or orange juice only. Take immediately after mixing.

- Loss of appetite
- Weight changes
- Drowsiness
- Dizziness
- Excessive tiredness
- Edema
- Decreased blood pressure
- Postural hypotension

Common Side Effects for the SSRIs as a Class

- Changes in alertness
- Decrease in libido and sexual arousal, and/or difficulty achieving orgasm
- Nausea
- Anxiety
- Headache
- Photosensitivity
- Tremor

Special Considerations

- Typically, SSRIs are started at a lower dose to see if the medication is tolerated. If the starting dose is tolerated after 1 to 2 weeks, then the antidepressant dose can be increased to the lower end of the usual dose range. That dose should be maintained for several weeks to determine if the dose is effective. At that point, the physician could then recommend a higher dose if necessary.
- Lower doses and increased time between adjustments should be used in patients with liver disease and over the age of 65.
- If either sleepiness or insomnia occurs, then the timing of taking the medication can be arranged to accommodate the change. If the medication makes the patient sleepy, then the medication can be taken at bedtime. If it causes the person to stay awake or experience insomnia, then the medication can be taken upon rising or early in the day.
- SSRIs can actually help treat anxiety. However, symptoms of anxiety have been reported when patients first start the drug but typically disappear once sustained on a usual dose. To avoid this side

effect the initial dose should be low, and the medication increased slowly. If a patient still reports anxious feelings, then discussion with the prescriber should take place to determine if the patient can tolerate it or if the drug should be discontinued.

- Some individuals experience the occurrence of feeling distant or not having a care along with an improved mood. Some call this the "Teflonization" from the SSRIs; a "What? Me worry?" sense of not caring that can change one's personality.
- Patients should avoid activities that require alertness and good coordination until the central nervous system (CNS) effects of the drug are known.
- Serotonin syndrome is a rare but potentially life-threatening syndrome characterized by symptoms such as increased fever, sweating, increased blood pressure, mental status changes, and increased reflexes. It can occur when two or more drugs are given simultaneously that dramatically increase serotonin for a sustained amount of time. Because people's bodies are different, some people may be more prone to develop this syndrome than others. To avoid serotonin syndrome it is recommended to wash out from one serotonin modulating agent before starting another. Drugs that could potentially interact with SSRIs and produce serotonin syndrome include:

  - MAOIs: phenelzine, isocarboxazid, tranylcypromine, and potentially, higher doses of selegiline and rasagiline
  - Meperidine
  - Fentanyl
  - Pentazocine
  - Tramadol
  - Ondansetron
  - Metoclopramide
  - Granisetron
  - Sumatriptan
  - Linezolid
  - Ritonavir
  - Dextromethorphan
  - Sibutramine

Please refer to drug reference guides for dose ranges and a complete list of drug interactions and adverse effects.

Paroxetine (PAXIL®)

Paroxetine is an antidepressant classified as SSRI (see Table 3.17).

Targets of therapy of paroxetine include:

- Depression
- Posttraumatic stress disorder
- Obsessive-compulsive disorder
- Panic disorder
- Premenstrual dysphoric disorder
- Social anxiety disorder

Side Effects

As with most medications, side effects may occur when treatment starts, when the dose is changed, or at any time; not everyone will experience side effects. Potential side effects include:

- Dizziness
- Weakness
- Difficulty concentrating
- Nervousness
- Confusion
- Vomiting
- Diarrhea
- Constipation
- Gas
- Stomach pain
- Heartburn
- Changes in ability to taste food
- Decreased appetite

Table 3.17

PAROXETINE (PAXIL®)	
Available as:	10 mg, 20 mg, 30 mg, 40 mg tablets 10 mg/5 mL oral suspension (orange flavored) 12.5 mg, 25 mg, 37.5 mg CR tablets

- Weight loss or gain
- Dry mouth
- Sweating
- Yawning
- Runny nose
- Cough
- Pain in the back, muscles, joints, or anywhere in the body
- Flushing
- Unusual dreams
- Painful or irregular menstruation

Common Side Effects for the SSRIs as a Class

- Changes in alertness
- Decrease in libido and sexual arousal, and/or difficulty achieving orgasm
- Nausea
- Anxiety
- Headache
- Photosensitivity

Special Considerations

- Typically, SSRIs are started at a lower dose to see if the medication is tolerated. If the starting dose is tolerated after 1 to 2 weeks, then the antidepressant dose can be increased to the lower end of the usual dose range. That dose should be maintained for several weeks to determine if the dose is effective. At that point, the physician could then recommend a higher dose if necessary.
- Lower doses and increased time between adjustments should be used in patients with liver disease and over the age of 65.
- If either sleepiness or insomnia should occur, then the timing of taking the medication can be arranged to accommodate the change. If the medication makes the patient sleepy, then the medication can be taken at bedtime. If it causes the person to stay awake or experience insomnia, then the medication can be taken upon rising or early in the day.
- SSRIs can actually help treat anxiety. However, symptoms of anxiety have been reported when patients first start the drug but typically disappear once sustained on a usual dose. To avoid this side

effect the initial dose should be low, and the medication increased slowly. If a patient still reports anxious feelings then discussion with the prescriber should take place to determine if the patient can tolerate it or if the drug should be discontinued.

- Some individuals experience the occurrence of feeling distant or not having a care along with an improved mood. Some call this the "Teflonization" from the SSRIs; a "What? Me worry?" sense of not caring that can change one's personality.
- Paroxetine affects histamine more than the other SSRIs, and taking it with medications for allergies classified as antihistamines may produce excessive sedation.
- Patients should avoid activities that require alertness and good coordination until the CNS effects of the drug are known.
- Serotonin syndrome is a rare but potentially fatal syndrome characterized by symptoms such as increased fever, sweating, increased blood pressure, mental status changes, and increased reflexes. It can occur when two or more drugs are given simultaneously that dramatically increase serotonin for a sustained amount of time. Because people's bodies are different, some people may be more prone to develop this syndrome than others. To avoid serotonin syndrome it is recommended to wash out from one serotonin modulating agent before starting another. Drugs that could potentially interact with SSRIs and produce serotonin syndrome include:
  - MAOIs: phenelzine, isocarboxazid, tranylcypromine, and potentially, higher doses of selegiline and rasagiline
  - Meperidine
  - Fentanyl
  - Pentazocine
  - Tramadol
  - Ondansetron
  - Metoclopramide
  - Granisetron
  - Sumatriptan
  - Linezolid
  - Ritonavir
  - Dextromethorphan
  - Sibutramine

Please refer to drug reference guides for dose ranges and a complete list of drug interactions and adverse effects.

Citalopram (CELEXA®)

Citalopram is an antidepressant classified as a selective serotonin reuptake inhibitor, SSRI. Citalopram is very selective in that it mostly affects serotonin only (see Table 3.18).

Targets of therapy of citalopram include:

- Depression

Side Effects

As with most medications, side effects may occur when treatment starts, when the dose is changed, or at any time; not everyone will experience side effects.

Potential side effects include:

- Diarrhea
- Constipation
- Vomiting
- Stomach pain
- Drowsiness
- Excitement
- Nervousness
- Muscle or joint pain
- Dry mouth

Common Side Effects for the SSRIs as a Class

- Changes in alertness
- Decrease in libido and/or sexual arousal, and/or difficulty achieving orgasm

Table 3.18

CITALOPRAM (CELEXA®)	
Available as:	10 mg, 20 mg, 40 mg tablet 10 mg/mL oral solution (peppermint flavored)

- Nausea
- Anxiety
- Headache
- Photosensitivity

Special Considerations

- Typically, SSRIs are started at a lower dose to see if the medication is tolerated. If the starting dose is tolerated after 1 to 2 weeks, then the antidepressant dose can be increased to the lower end of the usual dose range. That dose should be maintained for several weeks to determine if the dose is effective. At that point, the physician could recommend a higher dose if necessary.
- Lower doses and increased time between adjustments should be used in patients with liver disease and over the age of 65.
- If either sleepiness or insomnia occurs, then the timing of taking the medication can be altered to alleviate the side effect. For example, if the medication makes the patient sleepy, then the medication can be taken at bedtime. If it causes the person to stay awake or experience insomnia, then the medication can be taken upon rising or early in the day.
- SSRIs can actually help treat anxiety. However, symptoms of anxiety have been reported when patients first start the drug but typically disappear once sustained on a usual dose. To avoid this side effect the initial dose should be low, and the medication increased slowly. If a patient still reports anxious feelings, then discussion with the prescriber should take place to determine if the patient can tolerate it or if the drug should be discontinued.
- Some individuals experience the occurrence of feeling distant or not having a care along with an improved mood. Some call this the "Teflonization" from the SSRIs; a "What? Me worry?" sense of not caring that can change one's personality.
- Patients should avoid activities that require alertness and good coordination until the CNS effects of the drug are known.
- Serotonin syndrome is a rare but potentially fatal syndrome characterized by symptoms such as increased fever, sweating, increased blood pressure, mental status changes, and increased reflexes. It can potentially occur when two or more drugs are given simultaneously that dramatically increase serotonin for a sustained amount of

time. Because people's bodies are different, some people may be more prone to develop this syndrome than others. To avoid serotonin syndrome it is recommended to wash out from one serotonin modulating agent before starting another. Drugs that could potentially interact with SSRIs and produce serotonin syndrome include:

- MAOIs: phenelzine, isocarboxazid, tranylcypromine, and potentially, higher doses of selegiline and rasagiline
- Meperidine
- Fentanyl
- Pentazocine
- Tramadol
- Ondansetron
- Metoclopramide
- Granisetron
- Sumatriptan
- Linezolid
- Ritonavir
- Dextromethorphan
- Sibutramine

Please refer to drug reference guides for dose ranges and a complete list of drug interactions and adverse effects.

Escitalopram (LEXAPRO®)

Escitalopram is an antidepressant classified as an SSRI (see Table 3.19).

Targets of therapy of escitalopram include:

- Depression
- Generalized anxiety disorder

Table 3.19

ESCITALOPRAM (LEXAPRO®)	
Available as:	5 mg,10 mg, 20 mg tablet 5 mg/5 mL oral solution (peppermint flavored)

Side Effects

As with most medications, side effects may occur when treatment starts, when the dose is changed, or at any time; not everyone will experience side effects. Potential side effects include:

- Diarrhea
- Constipation
- Drowsiness
- Increased sweating
- Headache
- Stomach pain
- Dry mouth
- Increased appetite

Common Side Effects for the SSRIs as a Class

- Changes in alertness
- Decrease in libido and/or sexual arousal, and/or difficulty achieving orgasm
- Nausea
- Anxiety
- Headache
- Photosensitivity

Special Considerations

- Typically, SSRIs are started at a lower dose to see if the medication is tolerated. If the starting dose is tolerated after 1 to 2 weeks, then the antidepressant dose can be increased to the lower end of the usual dose range. That dose should be maintained for several weeks to determine if the dose is effective. At that point, the physician could recommend a higher dose if necessary.
- Lower doses and increased time between adjustments should be used in patients with liver disease and over the age of 65.
- If either sleepiness or insomnia occurs, then the timing of taking the medication can be altered to alleviate the side effect. For example, if the medication makes the patient sleepy, then the

medication can be taken at bedtime. If it causes the person to stay awake or experience insomnia, then the medication can be taken upon rising or early in the day.

- SSRIs can actually help treat anxiety. However, symptoms of anxiety have been reported when patients first start the drug but typically disappear once sustained on a usual dose. To avoid this side effect, the initial dose should be low, and the medication increased slowly. If a patient still reports anxious feelings, then discussion with the prescriber should take place to determine if the patient can tolerate it or if the drug should be discontinued.
- Some individuals experience the occurrence of feeling distant or not having a care along with an improved mood. Some call this the "Teflonization" from the SSRIs; a "What? Me worry?" sense of not caring that can change one's personality.
- Patients should avoid activities that require alertness and good coordination until the CNS effects of the drug are known.
- Serotonin syndrome is a rare but potentially fatal syndrome characterized by symptoms such as increased fever, sweating, increased blood pressure, mental status changes, and increased reflexes. It can potentially occur when two or more drugs are given simultaneously that dramatically increase serotonin for a sustained amount of time. Because people's bodies are different, some people may be more prone to develop this syndrome than others. To avoid serotonin syndrome it is recommended to wash out from one serotonin modulating agent before starting another. Drugs that could potentially interact with SSRIs and produce serotonin syndrome include:

    - MAOIs: phenelzine, isocarboxazid, tranylcypromine, and potentially, higher doses of selegiline and rasagiline
    - Meperidine
    - Fentanyl
    - Pentazocine
    - Tramadol
    - Ondansetron
    - Metoclopramide
    - Granisetron
    - Sumatriptan
    - Linezolid

- Ritonavir
- Dextromethorphan
- Sibutramine

Please refer to drug reference guides for dose ranges and a complete list of drug interactions and adverse effects.

OTHER AGENTS USED FOR DEPRESSION IN PARKINSON'S DISEASE

Bupropion (WELLBUTRIN®)

Bupropion is an agent used in the management of depression. Bupropion works mostly on dopamine, and it is also classified as a weak inhibitor of norepinephrine and serotonin. This antidepressant has more of an activating effect, and it is also used for chronic fatigue syndrome. It differs mechanistically from the SSRIs and anticholinergic medications; therefore, it also has less anticholinergic side effects (i.e., dry mouth, urinary retention, confusion, and constipation) associated with its use. Moreover, if the sexual side effects of SSRIs are an issue with the patient, the bupropion can either be added or used in its place.

Targets of therapy of bupropion include:

- Depression
- Chronic fatigue syndrome

Side Effects

As with most medications, side effects may occur when treatment starts, when the dose is changed, or at any time; not everyone will experience side effects. Potential side effects include:

- Agitation
- Constipation
- Dry mouth
- Headache
- Insomnia
- Nausea
- Vomiting

Table 3.20

BUPROPION (WELLBUTRIN®)
Available as: 75 mg and 100 mg tablets 100 mg, 150 mg, and 200 mg sustained release tablets 150 mg and 300 mg extended release tablets

- Tremor
- Dizziness
- Tachycardia
- Blurred vision
- Increased sweating
- Irritability
- Seizures

Special Considerations

- Do not use with the smoking cessation aid, Zyban®.
- If using bupropion in a patient on medication to treat Parkinson's disease, then the initial dose of bupropion should be low and increased very slowly.
- Patients with epilepsy or those prone to seizures should avoid this medication.
- Patients should avoid activities that require alertness and good coordination until the CNS effects of the drug are known (see Table 3.20).

Please refer to drug reference guides for dose ranges and a complete list of drug interactions and adverse effects.

Duloxetine (CYMBALTA®)

Duloxetine works on both serotonin and norepinephrine. Although similar to venla, duloxetine does affect norepinephrine at the lower doses.

Targets of therapy of duloxetine include:

- Depression
- Neuropathic pain associated with diabetes

Side Effects

As with most medications, side effects may occur when treatment starts, when the dose is changed, or at any time; not everyone will experience side effects. Potential side effects include:

- Dizziness
- Fatigue
- Somnolence
- Tremor
- Constipation
- Increased sweating
- Dry mouth
- Nausea
- Decreased appetite
- Blurred vision
- Sexual dysfunction

Special Considerations

- Antidepressant effects may take as long as 4–6 weeks until a full benefit is seen.
- It is not recommended that patients with severe renal impairment or liver dysfunction take this medication.
- Liver enzymes should be monitored while taking duloxetine.
- It is not recommended that alcohol be consumed because it may increase risk of liver toxicity.
- Patients should avoid activities that require alertness and good coordination until the CNS effects of the drug are known (see Table 3.21).

Table 3.21

DULOXETINE (CYMBALTA®)
Available as: 20 mg, 30 mg, and 60 mg delayed release capsules
The capsules are to be swallowed whole and not chewed, crushed, or sprinkled onto food.

Please refer to drug reference guides for dose ranges and a complete list of drug interactions and adverse effects.

Venlafaxine (EFFEXOR®)

Venlafaxine works on serotonin at lower doses and norepinephrine at higher doses. It is classified as an antidepressant, and may be useful in patients who do not respond to the SSRIs.

Targets of therapy of venlafaxine include:

- Depression
- Generalized anxiety disorder
- Social anxiety disorder

Side Effects

As with most medications, side effects may occur when treatment starts, when the dose is changed, or at any time; not everyone will experience side effects. Potential side effects include:

- Anxiety
- Dizziness
- Insomnia
- Nervousness
- Headache
- Nausea
- Increased sweating
- Abnormal ejaculation
- Appetite changes
- Constipation
- Tremor
- Blurred vision

Special Considerations

- When beginning treatment, it is important to begin with low doses and titrate up slowly as these agents may produce more anxiety when titrated up quickly.
- This medication should be taken with food.

Table 3.22

VENLAFAXINE (EFFEXOR®)
Available as: 25 mg, 37.5 mg, 50 mg, 75 mg, and 100 mg tablet 37.5 mg, 75 mg, and 150 mg extended release capsule
The capsules are to be swallowed whole and not chewed, crushed, or sprinkled onto food.

- In patients with renal or liver disease the dose should be reduced to 50% of the normal dose.
- Patients should avoid activities that require alertness and good coordination until the CNS effects of the drug are known (see Table 3.22).

Please refer to drug reference guides for dose ranges and a complete list of drug interactions and adverse effects.

Mirtazapine (REMERON®)

Mirtazapine has noradrenergic and serotonergic activity. Mirtazapine was first used as an antidepressant, but now it is also used as a sleeping aid and to increase appetite in some patients. Patients report symptom improvement as soon as 1–4 weeks after beginning treatment.

Targets of therapy of mirtazapine include:

- Depression
- Loss of appetite
- Insomnia

Side Effects

As with most medications, side effects may occur when treatment starts, when the dose is changed, or at any time; not everyone will experience side effects. Potential side effects include:

- Confusion
- Dizziness
- Somnolence

Table 3.23

MIRTAZAPINE (REMERON®)
Available as: 7.5 mg, 15 mg, 30 mg, and 45 mg tablets 15 mg, 30 mg, and 45 mg orally disintegrating tablets

- Constipation
- Increased appetite
- Weight gain
- Chest pain
- Tachycardia
- Postural hypotension

Special Considerations

- Cautious dosing should be used in patients who are elderly, have decreased renal function, or have decreased liver function.
- It is not recommended that alcohol be consumed with this medication because central nervous system side effects such as cognitive and motor impairment may be intensified.
- Patients should avoid activities that require alertness and good coordination until the CNS effects of the drug are known.
- Utilize lower doses when using for insomnia.
- Special caution should be exercised when taking this medication in conjunction with rasagiline.
- There are reports that conditions such as restless legs syndrome are either new onset or are exacerbated by mirtazapine.
- Advise patients to contact their physician immediately if flulike symptoms develop, because there are rare cases of mirtazapine causing agranulocytosis (see Table 3.23).

Please refer to drug reference guides for dose ranges and a complete list of drug interactions and adverse effects.

Trazodone (DESYREL®)

Trazodone is primarily used for insomnia; particularly it is helpful to help individuals fall asleep as well as to lessen the occurrence of early morning awakenings. Trazodone is classified as a serotonin-adrenergic reuptake inhibitor. The agent has weak agonist/antagonist properties on serotonin receptors. It also mildly blocks adrenergic receptors. It has mild antidepressant properties, but often requires much higher doses to achieve this effect. Therefore, it is usually not the first-line choice for treatment of depression as SSRIs are now available.

Side Effects

As with most medications, side effects may occur when treatment starts, when the dose is changed, or at any time; not everyone will experience side effects. Potential side effects include:

- Changes in blood pressure
- Dizziness
- Confusion
- Drowsiness
- Headache
- Uncoordination
- Tremors
- Dry mouth
- Blurred vision
- Weight gain
- Urinary retention
- Priapism (prolonged and painful erection)

Special Considerations

- This medication should be taken with food to decrease dizziness and orthostatic hypotension.

Table 3.24

TRAZODONE (DESYREL®)
Available as: 50 mg, 100 mg, 150 mg, 300 mg tablets

- It is not advisable to take trazodone with alcohol because of the increased risks of central nervous system side effects and sedation.
- Patients should avoid activities that require alertness and good coordination until the CNS effects of the drug are known.
- The prescribing doctor may want to consider more conservative dosing in the elderly because trazodone can be very sedating (see Table 3.24).

Please refer to drug reference guides for dose ranges and a complete list of drug interactions and adverse effects.

Tricyclic Antidepressants (TCA)

Examples include:

Amitriptyline (ELAVIL®)

Imipramine (TOFRANIL®)

Doxepin (SINEQUAN®)

TCAs may be beneficial in patients with insomnia, bladder hyperactivity, and drooling, because of their anticholinergic effects (see Tables 3.25 and 3.26). In contrast, these anticholinergic properties may worsen cognitive impairment, hallucinations, hypotension, or excessive daytime somnolence. Depressed patients with comorbid anxiety may also respond better to SSRIs.

Table 3.25

TRICYCLIC ANTIDEPRESSANTS

Amitriptyline (Elavil®)
Available as: 25 mg, 50 mg, 75 mg, 100 mg, 150 mg tablets

Imipramine (Tofranil®)
Available as: 10 mg, 25 mg, 50 mg tablets

Doxepin
Available as: 10 mg, 25 mg, 50 mg, 75 mg, 100 mg tablets

Table 3.26

SIDE EFFECTS OF ANTIDEPRESSANTS USED IN PD

DRUG	DOSE (MG/DAY)	SEDATION	HYPOTENSION	ANTIMUSCARINIC EFFECTS	SEXUAL DYSFUNCTION	WEIGHT GAIN
Fluoxetine	10 to 80	+/–	+/–	+/–	+++	+
Fluvoxamine	50 to 300	+/	+/–	+/–	++	++
Paroxetine	20 to 50	+	+/	+	+++	++
Sertraline	25 to 100	+/–	+/	+/–	++	+
Citalopram	10 to 60	+	+/	+	++	+
Escitalopram	10 to 20	+	+/	+	++	+
Amitriptyline	25 to 200	+++	++	+++	+	+++
Doxepin	75 to 150	++	++	+++	+	++
Imipramine	50 to 200	++	+++	++	+	++
Desipramine	100 to 300	+	+	+	+/	+
Nortriptyline	50 to 150	+	+	+	+/	+
Bupropion	150 to 450	+/–	+/–	+	+/	+/–
Mirtazapine	15 to 45	++	++	+	++	+++
Nefazodone	300 to 600	++	++	+/–	+	+/–
Venlafaxine	75 to 375	+	+/–	+	+++	+

+/– = minimal or negligible; + = mild; ++ = moderate; +++ = considerable

Side Effects

TCAs have common side effects, which include:

- Dry mouth
- Drowsiness
- Constipation
- Blurred vision
- Urinary hesitancy; incontinence
- Memory loss and cognitive slowing
- Confusion
- Hypotension; orthostasis; fainting
- Heart rhythm problems
- Sexual problems
- Weight gain

Special Considerations

- Caution must be used when prescribing this class of agents with MAO inhibitors such as rasagiline.
- This class of drugs is best avoided in the elderly, especially those with cognitive impairment, heart rhythm problems, and prostate enlargement.
- They are best used at night because of their strong sedative effects.
- It is best to start at very low doses and increase slowly for better tolerability.
- These drugs should also be avoided in patients with glaucoma or increased intraocular pressure.

ANTIPSYCHOTIC AGENTS BEST TOLERATED IN PARKINSON'S DISEASE

Clozapine (CLOZARIL®, FAZACLO®)

Hallucinations and delusions can occur in patients with Parkinson's disease. This is usually due to anti-Parkinson drug side effects. If, despite reducing or stopping unnecessary medications, the patient is still experiencing hallucinations, then it may be appropriate to use an antipsychotic medication.

Table 3.27

CLOZAPINE	
Clozaril® Available as: 25 mg, 100 mg tablets	**FazaClo®** Orally disintegrating tablet: 25 mg, 100 mg

Clozapine is an atypical antipsychotic, which has been shown to be effective in patients with PD and psychosis while not worsening the motor features of PD (see Table 3.27). Although clozapine may provide the best results as compared to other atypical antipsychotics, its use is limited by the potential of serious side effects; particularly agranulocytosis. A patient registry and monitoring system is in place to monitor white blood counts (see below). Other potential serious side effects, although rare, include seizures (usually at higher dosages), orthostatic hypotension, syncope, and myocarditis.

Side Effects

As with most medications, side effects may occur when treatment starts, when the dose is changed, or at any time; not everyone will experience side effects. Potential side effects include:

- Excess saliva
- Sedation
- Orthostatic hypotension
- Weight gain
- Dizziness
- Constipation
- Tachycardia
- Hyperglycemia
- Nausea
- Vomiting
- Confusion
- Decreased libido

Although rare, more serious side effects include:

- Agranulocytosis
- Seizures
- Myocarditis
- Neuroleptic malignant syndrome
- Syncope

Special Considerations

- Clozapine has been reported to cause significant bone marrow suppression resulting in agranulocytosis where deaths have been reported.
- It is important that the patient be informed about agranulocytosis and how it is managed. The importance of keeping all doctor visits should be emphasized.
- Clozapine administration initially requires weekly complete blood count (CBC) with differential to monitor for agranulocytosis.
- The absolute neutrophil count (ANC) can be calculated by multiplying the total white blood cell (WBC) count by the percent of neutrophils.
- Percent of neutrophils is the sum of the percent of segmented neutrophils plus the percent of bands.
- Acceptable dispensing values are WBC counts ≥3,000/mm^3 and ANCs ≥1,500/mm^3.
- A WBC count <3,500/mm^3 or an ANC <2,000/mm^3 is an indication of leukopenia or granulocytopenia, and patients should be monitored closely.
- Frequency of monitoring is based on stage of therapy or results from WBC count and ANC monitoring tests.
- Initiation of therapy and WBC and ANC monitoring is obtained weekly for 6 months as long as hematologic values for monitoring are WBC ≥3,500/mm^3, ANC ≥2,000/mm^3.
- If all results for WBC ≥3,500/mm^3, and ANC ≥2,000/mm^3, after 6 months of therapy, monitoring between 6 months and 12 months of therapy can be performed every 2 weeks for 6 months.
- If all results for WBC ≥3,500/mm^3, and ANC ≥2,000/mm^3 after 12 months of therapy, monitoring can be extended to every 4 weeks indefinitely. At discontinuation of therapy, WBC and ANC monitoring should occur weekly for at least 4 weeks from day of discontinuation or until WBC ≥3,500/mm^3 and ANC ≥2,000/mm^3.

- If there is a single drop or cumulative drop within 3 weeks of WBC ≥ 3,000/mm^3 or ANC ≥ 1,500/mm^3, repeat WBC and ANC. If repeat values are 3,000/mm^3 < WBC < 3,500/mm^3 and ANC > 2,000/mm^3, then monitor twice weekly.
- If there is mild leukopenia, 3,500/mm^3 > WBC > 3,000/mm^3 and/or mild granulocytopenia, 2,000/mm^3 > ANC > 1,500/mm^3, perform twice-weekly monitoring until WBC > 3,500/mm^3 and ANC > 2,000/mm^3; then return to previous monitoring frequency.
- There is a warning associated with clozapine's use in the geriatric population, stating there is a risk of increased sudden cardiac death in elderly patients with dementia-related psychosis when compared to a placebo.

Please refer to drug reference guides for dose ranges and a complete list of drug interactions and adverse effects.

Quetiapine (SEROQUEL®)

Hallucinations and delusions can occur in patients with Parkinson's disease. This is usually due to anti-Parkinson drug side effects. If, despite reducing or stopping unnecessary medications, the patient is still experiencing hallucinations, then it may be appropriate to use an antipsychotic medication.

Quetiapine is an atypical antipsychotic used to reduce hallucinations without dramatically worsening the motor symptoms of Parkinson's disease (see Table 3.28). In addition it often improves sleep. Quetiapine is started in a low dose of one 25-mg tablet taken at bedtime because it can cause sleepiness. Typically, it is recommended to raise the dose by 25-mg (one tablet) increments every week until the hallucinations are controlled. For those with Parkinson's disease, low total daily doses of 25–100 mg daily are usually sufficient.

Table 3.28

QUETIAPINE (SEROQUEL®)
Available as: 25 mg, 100 mg, 150 mg, 200 mg tablets

Side Effects

As with most medications, side effects may occur when treatment starts, when the dose is changed, or at any time; not everyone will experience side effects. Potential side effects include:

- Sedation
- Postural hypotension
- Syncope
- Dizziness
- Agitation
- Weakness
- Nausea
- Vomiting
- Constipation
- Headache
- Weight gain
- Thinning of hair or nails
- Dry mouth

Special Considerations

- Quetiapine should be used with caution in patients with known cardiovascular disease, cerebrovascular disease, or other conditions predisposing to hypotension.
- Quetiapine may induce a drop in blood pressure on standing or sitting, especially during the initial dose-titration. Blood pressure and pulse should be recorded both lying and standing.
- A warning for all atypical antipsychotics has been given because of the unclear etiology of a slight increase in mortality among cognitively impaired patients taking these types of medications.
- Rarely, quetiapine may worsen parkinsonism, but this worsening is usually mild compared to other antipsychotic agents.
- Atypical antipsychotic agents have been reported to cause or worsen diabetes, although this remains to be confirmed in larger studies.

Please refer to drug reference guides for dose ranges and a complete list of drug interactions and adverse effects.

ANXIOLYTIC AGENTS USED IN PARKINSON'S DISEASE

Benzodiazepines

Benzodiazepines are a class of medications that may be useful in treating anxiety, insomnia, muscle stiffness, and seizures (see Table 3.29). Their use in Parkinson's disease is primarily related to their ability to help anxiety and insomnia. In addition, they have been reported to alleviate internal tremor, a feature in PD that is often associated with anxiety. They are typically used for brief periods of time, but sometimes are used chronically. Other types of medications such as antidepressants that have antianxiety properties are often more appropriate for the control of chronic anxiety.

Table 3.29

BENZODIAZEPINES

DRUG NAME	AVAILABLE STRENGTHS	COMMENTS
Alprazolam (Xanax®)	0.25, 0.5, 1, 2 mg tabs XR: 1.5, 1, 2, or 3 mg Oral solution 1 mg/mL	CYP3A4 drug interactions XR forms may be helpful in anxiety pts needing multiple daily dosing
Clonazepam (Klonopin®)	0.5 mg, 1 mg, 2 mg tabs Orally disintegrating: 0.125 mg, 0.25 mg, 0.5 mg, 1 mg, 2 mg	Caution in impaired renal function
Triazolam (Halcion®)	0.125 mg and 0.25 mg tabs	Tolerance may develop
Diazepam (Valium®)	2, 5, 10 mg tabs Oral solution: 5 mg/mL	Concentrated solution—mix with other liquids
Flurazepam (Dalmane®)	15, 30 mg caps	Avoid in elderly due to long half life
Lorazepam (Ativan®)	0.5, 1, 2 mg tabs Oral solution: 2 mg/mL	Better choice in liver disease
Oxazepam (Serax®)	15 mg caps 10, 15, 30 mg tabs	Better choice in liver disease
Quazepam (Doral®)	7.5, 15 mg tabs	
Temazepam (Restoril®)	7.5, 15, 30 mg caps	Better choice in liver disease

Benzodiazepines bind to GABA receptors in the central nervous system. GABA is a neurotransmitter that inhibits or blocks brain signaling. By binding to GABA receptors, benzodiazepines increase the effects of this inhibitory neurotransmitter, which as a result suppresses some brain activity and therefore is sedating and alleviates anxiety.

The effects of benzodiazepines differ from agent to agent, but generally these agents take effect within 30 minutes to 2 hours.

Side Effects

May differ from agent to agent but generally include:

- Drowsiness
- Dizziness
- Changes in heart rate
- Confusion (especially in elderly population)
- Changes in appetite
- Vomiting
- Nausea
- Changes in libido
- Urinary retention
- Visual disturbances (double vision, nystagmus)
- Psychosis
- Changes in behavior
- Hepatic dysfunction
- Increased fall risk

Symptoms of overdose include:

- Impaired coordination
- Diminished reflexes
- Respiratory depression
- Hypotension
- Hypotonia
- Coma

Special Considerations

- May cause drowsiness, so avoid driving or other tasks requiring alertness.

- It is not recommended to take these agents with alcohol because of the risk of experiencing central nervous system side effects such as drowsiness and dizziness.
- Individuals on long-term or high-dose treatment are at risk for experiencing withdrawal symptoms. In this case the physician should individualize dose titration off of the drug.

AGENTS USED FOR COGNITIVE PROBLEMS IN PARKINSON'S DISEASE

Donepezil (ARICEPT®)

Donepezil is an acetylcholinesterase inhibitor approved for mild, moderate, and severe Alzheimer's disease (see Table 3.30). Acetylcholinesterase is an enzyme that destroys acetylcholine, a chemical important for memory and cognitive function. By blocking the enzyme that breaks down acetylcholine, donepezil increases the available acetylcholine in the brain, thereby preserving cognitive functions. It has been studied in patients with Parkinson's disease who experience decreased cognition and memory impairment. Outcomes associated with donepezil include improved memory, psychomotor speed, and attention. While it is in the same class as rivastigmine, it is not yet FDA approved in the United States for use in Parkinson's disease.

Targets of therapy of donepezil include:

- Memory impairment
- Decreased psychomotor speed
- Decreased attention

Side Effects

As with most medications, side effects may occur when treatment starts, when the dose is changed, or at any time; not everyone will experience side effects. Potential side effects include:

- Nausea
- Vomiting
- Dizziness
- Diarrhea

Table 3.30

DONEPEZIL (ARICEPT®)
Available as: 5 mg and 10 mg tablets 5 mg and 10 mg orally disintegrating tablets

- Anorexia
- Headache
- Paranoia
- Agitation
- Irritability
- Vivid or abnormal dreams
- Tremor worsening

Special Considerations

- The dose is normally prescribed at bedtime; however, if the patient experiences vivid dreams that are bothersome, the dose may be taken in the morning.
- The orally disintegrating tablets should be dissolved on the tongue, then followed by a glass of water.
- Monitor patients with a history of gastrointestinal (GI) bleeding or patients concomitantly taking nonsteroidal anti-inflammatory drugs (NSAIDs). There have been reports of GI bleeding with donepezil.

Please refer to drug reference guides for dose ranges and a complete list of drug interactions and adverse effects.

Galantamine (RAZADYNE®)

Galantamine is a competitive and reversible inhibitor of acetylcholinesterase (see Table 3.31). It enhances cholinergic function by allowing concentrations of acetylcholine to increase and possibly allowing cholinergic neurons to stay intact. It is not as well studied as rivastigmine or donepezil, but it may be considered as a treatment option for patients in which other acetylcholinesterase drugs are contraindicated.

Table 3.31

GALANTAMINE (RAZADYNE®)
Available as: 4 mg, 8 mg, 12 mg immediate release tablets 8 mg, 16 mg, and 24 mg extended release tablets 4 mg/mL oral solution

Targets of therapy of galantamine include:

- Mild to moderate cognitive and memory impairments

Side Effects

As with most medications, side effects may occur when treatment starts, when the dose is changed, or at any time; not everyone will experience side effects. Potential side effects include:

- Nausea
- Dizziness
- Vomiting
- Anorexia
- Diarrhea
- Syncope
- Weight loss
- Depression
- Insomnia
- Somnolence
- Worsening of tremor
- Dyspepsia
- Abdominal pain
- Tremor worsening

Special Considerations

- Patients should contact the physician immediately if any of the following occur: severe nausea, vomiting, GI cramping, salivation, lacrimation, muscle weakness/fasciculations, or respiratory depression.

- GI symptoms can be reduced by taking galantamine with meals or concomitantly taking an antiemetic.
- Galantamine is usually prescribed twice daily and should be taken with the morning and evening meal.

Please refer to drug reference guides for dose ranges and a complete list of drug interactions and adverse effects.

Memantine (NAMENDA®)

Memantine is an agent approved for moderate to severe Alzheimer's and moderate to severe dementia (see Table 3.32). Memantine inhibits receptors in the brain known as N-methyl-D-aspartate (NMDA) from a neurotransmitter known as glutamate. In Alzheimer's and possibly Parkinson's disease these receptors may get overstimulated by glutamate. This overstimulation may decrease cognition. Memantine ultimately decreases glutamate release, allowing preservation of certain brain cells. This agent is currently not approved for Parkinson's disease dementia.

Targets of therapy of memantine include:

- Moderate to severe dementia

Side Effects

As with most medications, side effects may occur when treatment starts, when the dose is changed, or at any time; not everyone will experience side effects. Potential side effects include:

- Constipation
- Headache

Table 3.32

MEMANTINE (NAMENDA®)
Available as: 5 mg and 10 mg tablets (dosing titration packs are available); also available as a 2 m/mL solution

- Dizziness
- Increased blood pressure
- Mental status changes

Special Considerations

- During the first week of treatment there may be increased confusion observed with this drug. The patient/family should contact the health care provider if it is severe or does not decrease within a week.
- Use caution when the patient is on other NMDA antagonists such as amantadine, ketamine, and dextromethorphan.
- Psychosis has occurred in some individuals with Parkinson's disease using memantine.

Please refer to drug reference guides for dose ranges and a complete list of drug interactions and adverse effects.

Rivastigmine (EXELON®)

Some patients with Parkinson's disease may develop cognitive difficulties such as decreased attention, difficulty with memory retrieval (slowness in remembering words or names, for example), and impairment of *executive functions* (e.g., planning tasks, keeping track of things, and handling complex tasks). Rivastigmine is the only medication currently approved by the FDA for mild to moderate cognitive difficulties in PD (see Table 3.33). Rivastigmine is an acetylcholinesterase inhibitor. Acetylcholinesterase is an enzyme that destroys acetylcholine, a chemical important for memory and cognitive function. By blocking the enzyme that breaks down acetylcholine, rivastigmine increases the available acetylcholine in the brain, thereby preserving cognitive functions. Outcomes associated with this drug include improved memory, psychomotor speed, and attention.

A controlled study published in 2004 showed that rivastigmine has some benefits for those with PD. The study included patients over the age of 50, who had a Mini-Mental State Examination (MMSE) score of 10 to 24 (the MMSE is a standardized test of cognitive function with a perfect score of 30). The study showed a significant improvement in the PD patients on rivastigmine compared to patients on placebo, lasting at least 6 months in 60% of the study participants.

Table 3.33

RIVASTIGMINE	
Rivastigmine (Exelon®) Available as: 1.5 mg, 3 mg, 4.5 mg, 6 mg tablet Also available in a 2 mg/mL solution	**Rivastigmine transdermal system (Exelon Patch®)** Available as: 4.6 mg/24 hour transdermal patch and 9.5 mg/24 hour transdermal patch

More recently, 541 demented PD patients were enrolled in a double-blind study comparing rivastigminc versus placebo. The rivastigmine-treated patients had a mean improvement of 2.1 points in the Alzheimer's Disease Assessment Scale-cognitive subscale (ADAS-cog) compared to a 0.7 point worsening in the placebo group. This was the pivotal trial that led to the FDA approval of this drug for use in the PD population.

Targets of therapy of rivastigmine include:

- Mild to moderate dementia associated with Parkinson's disease
- Mild to moderate dementia of Alzheimer type

Side Effects

As with most medications, side effects may occur when treatment starts, when the dose is changed, or at any time; not everyone will experience side effects. Potential side effects include:

- Nausea
- Vomiting
- Anorexia
- Diarrhea
- Weight loss
- Bradycardia
- Urinary retention
- Insomnia
- Anxiety
- Hallucinations
- Somnolence

- Syncope
- Tremor worsening

Special Considerations

- Individuals should take this medication with food to decrease nausea and vomiting.
- Monitor patient's weight, and instruct patient to report weight loss.
- Use with caution in patients with asthma and COPD.
- Use with caution in patients with an active or history of gastrointestinal bleed/ulcer. Rivastigmine may increase gastric acid secretion, therefore increasing the risk of gastrointestinal bleeding.
- Because of its cholinergic nature, rivastigmine may worsen tremors. However, these are mostly mild and transient.
- Larger clinical trials do not show a significant worsening of other parkinsonian symptoms.

Please refer to drug reference guides for dose ranges and a complete list of drug interactions and adverse effects.

AGENTS USED FOR DYSTONIA

Botulinum Toxin, Type A (BOTOX®, DYSPORT®), Botulinum Toxin, Type B (MYOBLOC®)

Botulinum toxin is used primarily to treat the symptom of dystonia, which can be experienced by Parkinson patients. Dystonia is defined as a sustained or prolonged contraction of a muscle or group of muscles that results in abnormal posturing of the affected body part. In PD, the body parts most affected include the eyelids, hand, or foot, as well as the neck. Occasionally, other body parts such as the abdominal muscles can become dystonic, resulting in significant pain. Dystonia can occur from too much anti-Parkinson medication "peak dose" or too little when the person is wearing off or in an "off" state. Individuals diagnosed below the age of 40 are often more troubled by dystonia, which can sometimes be very painful. Other indications of botulinum toxin injection in PD include excessive sialorrhea (drooling) and diaphoresis (sweating). There have been a few reports of botulinum toxin injection relieving gait freezing.

Botulinum toxin works by blocking the release of acetylcholine at the neuromuscular junction. It is administered by injection into the affected muscle. Electromyography guidance is used depending on the muscles involved. Although expensive, this treatment has significantly improved functional status and quality of life for many individuals. The duration of action is approximately three to four months, and patients receive injections approximately three to four times a year.

Side Effects

- Muscle weakness beyond the desired effect
- Bruising at the injection site
- Allergic skin rash
- Flulike symptoms

Special Considerations

- Botulinum toxin should be administered by a physician specially trained in this treatment.

AGENTS COMMONLY USED FOR GASTROINTESTINAL DISTURBANCES

Lubiprostone (AMITIZA®)

Lubiprostone is indicated for chronic idiopathic constipation disease (see Table 3.34). This agent works to increase intestinal fluid secretion and gastric motility, facilitating stool passage.

Table 3.34

LUBIPROSTONE (AMITIZA®)
Available as: 8 mcg and 24 mcg capsules

Targets of therapy of lubiprostone include:

- Chronic idiopathic constipation
- Irritable bowel syndrome with constipation

Side Effects

As with most medications, side effects may occur when treatment starts, when the dose is changed, or at any time; not everyone will experience side effects. Potential side effects include:

- Nausea
- Diarrhea
- Headache
- Abdominal pain
- Tremor
- Anxiety
- Dyspnea
- Decreased appetite

Special Considerations

- Lubiprostone is used twice daily and should be taken with food.
- To prevent dehydration, the patient should drink 6–8 glasses of water per day.
- Lubiprostone should not be used in individuals with nausea because it increases risk of nausea.
- Patient/family should be instructed on nonpharmacological approaches to constipation including diet, exercise, establishing regular bowel routines, and increasing fluid intake.

Please refer to drug reference guides for dose ranges and a complete list of drug interactions and adverse effects.

Polyethylene Glycol (PEG) (MIRALAX®)

Polyethylene glycol is an agent that is used to treat constipation as commonly seen in Parkinson's disease (see Table 3.35). This laxative works by drawing water into the stool.

Table 3.35

POLYETHYLENE GLYCOL (PEG) (MIRALAX®)
Available as: 17 gram powder for oral solution

Target of therapy of polyethylene glycol include:

- Constipation

Side Effects

As with most medications, side effects may occur when treatment starts, when the dose is changed, or at any time; not everyone will experience side effects. Potential side effects include:

- Urticaria
- Nausea
- Abdominal bloating
- Cramping
- Flatulence
- Diarrhea

Special Considerations

- Usual dose is 17 grams of powder per day dissolved in 8 ounces of water.
- It is not recommended that this agent be used longer than 2 weeks.
- Reconstituted solution should be refrigerated and is good for 48 hours.
- Advise patients to not eat solid foods 3–4 hours before dosing.
- This agent should not be used in patients with a known or suspected bowel obstruction.
- If excessive, stool frequency may lead to an electrolyte imbalance, and if excessive stool frequency is noticed, the doctor should be contacted.

- Patient/family should be instructed on nonpharmacological approaches to constipation including diet, exercise, establishing regular bowel routines, and increasing fluid intake.

Please refer to drug reference guides for dose ranges and a complete list of drug interactions and adverse effects.

Senna (SENAKOT®)

Sennosides are derived from a plant and are classified as stimulant laxatives (see Table 3.36). They work by stimulating contractions, known as peristalsis, in the intestine by working directly on the intestinal mucosa. Following administration, a bowel movement will usually occur in 6–24 hours.

Targets of therapy of senna include:

- Constipation

Side Effects

As with most medications, side effects may occur when treatment starts, when the dose is changed, or at any time; not everyone will experience side effects. Potential side effects include:

- Diarrhea
- Nausea
- Vomiting
- Perianal irritation
- Fainting
- Bloating

Table 3.36

SENNA (SENAKOT®)
Available as tablets, granules, suppositories, and syrups in several strengths

- Flatulence
- Cramps
- Urine discoloration

Special Considerations

- Usual dose is 2–4 tablets once or twice daily. It is not recommended that dosage exceed 4 tablets twice daily.
- Patient should be instructed to take with a full glass of water.
- Excessive use may lead to an electrolyte imbalance.
- Patient/family should be instructed on nonpharmacological approaches to constipation including diet, exercise, establishing regular bowel routines, and increasing fluid intake.

Please refer to drug reference guides for dose ranges and a complete list of drug interactions and adverse effects.

AGENTS USED FOR SKIN CONDITIONS IN PARKINSON'S DISEASE

Betamethasone Valerate and Betamethasone Dipropionate

Betamethasone is a topical corticosteroid indicated in the treatment of skin conditions marked by inflammation and itching (see Table 3.37). Betamethasone is absorbed through the skin, where it then possesses

Table 3.37

BETAMETHASONE	
Betamethasone valerate	**Betamethasone dipropionate**
Available as topical application	Available for topical application
0.01% ointment	0.05% ointment
0.05% cream	0.05% cream
0.1% cream	0.05% lotion
0.1% lotion	0.01% aerosol
1.2 mg/g foam	

anti-inflammatory, antipruritic, and vasoconstrictive properties to help alleviate various skin conditions. It is used to treat seborrheic dermatitis in individuals with Parkinson's disease.

Targets of therapy of betamethasone include:

- Inflammatory skin conditions
- Pruritus

Side Effects

As with most medications, side effects may occur when treatment starts, when the dose is changed, or at any time; not everyone will experience side effects. Potential side effects include local site reactions that are generally mild and may include:

- Burning
- Itching
- Stinging

Additional potential adverse effects include:

- Striae (stretch marks)
- Hypothalamic-Pituitary-Adrenal (HPA) axis suppression
- Skin atrophy
- Secondary infection
- Hair loss
- Glycosuria with dipropionate

Special Considerations

- Systemic absorption can produce a Cushing's diseaselike state marked by increased blood glucose levels. This is reversible upon discontinuing the drug. Risk factors include using a higher potency steroid, using the product over large areas, prolonged use, and using occlusive dressing.
- When using cream and ointment, a thin layer should be applied 1 to 2 times daily.
- When using lotions shake well, and apply a few drops and rub in gently twice daily. Once condition begins improving, then dose once daily.

- When using foam, invert the can, apply a small amount in a cool container, pick up a small amount with the fingers, and massage gently into scalp. May be used twice daily.
- Do not use an occlusive dressing.

Please refer to drug reference guides for dose ranges and a complete list of drug interactions and adverse effects.

Fluocinolone Topical (CAPEX® Shampoo)

Fluocinolone is a topical corticosteroid which has low to medium potency (see Table 3.38). Because it is a topical corticosteroid it has anti-inflammatory, antipruritic, and vasoconstrictive properties.

Targets of therapy of fluocinolone topical include:

- Atopic dermatitis
- Psoriasis
- Seborrheic dermatitis of the scalp

Side Effects

As with most medications, side effects may occur when treatment starts, when the dose is changed, or at any time; not everyone will experience side effects. Potential side effects include:

- Dryness
- Foliculitis
- Acne
- Hypopigmentation
- Secondary skin infection
- Skin atrophy

Table 3.38

FLUOCINOLONE TOPICAL (CAPEX® SHAMPOO)
Available as a 0.01% shampoo which the pharmacist must mix prior to dispensing

- Burning
- Itching
- Irritation

Special Considerations

- Patients receiving other corticosteroids should only be treated with Capex® for only 2 weeks at a time.
- Shake well before using.
- No more than 1 ounce of shampoo should be applied to the scalp once daily.
- The product should be worked into the scalp and allowed to sit for about 5 minutes.
- After about 5 minutes, thoroughly wash hair and scalp with water.
- Do not use an occlusive dressing.
- Contents should be discarded after 3 months.

Please refer to drug reference guides for dose ranges and a complete list of drug interactions and adverse effects.

Hydrocortisone Topical

Hydrocortisone is a topical corticosteroid with anti-inflammatory, antipruritic, and vasoconstrictive properties (see Table 3.39). It is available over the counter to treat conditions such as poison ivy, insect bites, eczema, and any other irritation that is associated with itching or inflamma-

Table 3.39

HYDROCORTISONE TOPICAL (OVER THE COUNTER)	
Available as:	0.5%, 1%, and 2.5% ointment
	0.5%, 1%, and 2.5% cream
	1%, 2%, 2.5% lotion
	1% liquid
	1% and 2 % gel
	1% and 2.5% solution
	1% spray
	1% stick, roll on

tion. Individuals with Parkinson's disease may find this agent beneficial in treating seborrheic dermatitis.

Targets of therapy of topical hydrocortisone include:

- Inflammatory skin conditions
- Pruritus

Side Effects

As with most medications, side effects may occur when treatment starts, when the dose is changed, or at any time; not everyone will experience side effects. Potential side effects include:

- Stinging or burning on sensitive areas
- Irritation
- Dryness
- Hypopigmentation
- Secondary infection
- Skin atrophy
- Striae (stretch marks)

Special Considerations

- Generally a thin layer is applied to the affected area 2 to 4 times daily depending on the severity of the condition.
- Occlusive dressing may be used, but if signs and symptoms of an infection develop, the occlusive dressing should be discontinued and the health care provider contacted.
- If condition does not improve after 7 days, the health care provider should be consulted.
- Any strength greater than 1% is available by prescription only.

Please refer to drug reference guides for dose ranges and a complete list of drug interactions and adverse effects.

Ketoconazole (NIZORAL®)

Ketoconazole is a broad-spectrum antifungal agent (see Table 3.40). Ketoconazole cream is used for various fungal infections such as athlete's

Table 3.40

KETOCONAZOLE		
Ketoconazole 15 gm, 30 gm, and 60 gm 2% cream	**Nizoral®** 1% and 2% shampoo	**Xolegel®** 15 gram 2% gel

foot. However, the gel formulation and especially the shampoo formulation are beneficial in individuals with PD who have seborrheic dermatitis. The shampoo specifically may help decrease scaling associated with dandruff.

Targets of therapy of topical ketoconazole include:

- Fungal infections
- Seborrheic dermatitis

Side Effects

As with most medications, side effects may occur when treatment starts, when the dose is changed, or at any time; not everyone will experience side effects. Potential side effects include:

- Hair loss
- Irritation
- Abnormal hair texture
- Scalp pustules
- Dryness or oiliness of hair and scalp
- Itching

Special Considerations

- A sufficient amount of shampoo should be applied to wet hair (enough to lather).
- Gently massage over entire scalp for about 1 minute.
- Rinse hair thoroughly with warm water.
- Repeat process, leaving the treatment on the scalp for 3 more minutes.
- Scalp should be shampooed twice a week for 4 weeks.

- Separate each shampooing by at least 3 days.
- Potential drug interactions include: cisapride, dofetilide, eplerenone, ergoloid mesylates, pimozide, ranolazine, terfenadine, triazolam, aprepitant, alosetron, erythromycin, midazolam, fentanyl, sirolimus, fosamprenavir, lopinavir.

Please refer to drug reference guides for dose ranges and a complete list of drug interactions and adverse effects.

Pimecrolimus Topical (ELIDEL®)

Pimecrolimus is a calcineurin inhibitor (see Table 3.41). It inhibits key molecules that predispose an allergic reaction. Pimecrolimus is generally used in the treatment of mild to moderate atopic dermatitis when other agents have failed.

Targets of therapy pimecrolimus include:

- Atopic dermatitis

Side Effects

As with most medications, side effects may occur when treatment starts, when the dose is changed, or at any time; not everyone will experience side effects. Potential side effects include:

- Secondary infection
- Burning, itching, redness of application site
- Headache
- Acne
- Diarrhea
- Nausea
- Vomiting

Table 3.41

PIMECROLIMUS TOPICAL (ELIDEL®)
Available as a 1% cream in 30, 60, and 100 gram tubes

Special Considerations

- Apply a thin layer to affected skin twice daily.
- Stop use when signs and symptoms resolve.
- Do not bathe, shower, or swim immediately following application.
- Do not cover with an occlusive dressing.
- Application should be limited to a small area and used only for a short term. Long-term safety is unknown.
- Exposure to natural and artificial sunlight should be minimized while on this agent.
- Avoid this agent in immuno-compromised individuals.
- Potential for drug interaction exists with erythromycin, itraconazole, ketoconazole, fluconazole, calcium channel blockers, cimetadine.

Please refer to drug reference guides for dose ranges and a complete list of drug interactions and adverse effects.

Salicylic Acid/Sulfur Topical (SEBULEX® Shampoo)

Salicylic acid is available over the counter and in many different formulations; however, the shampoo formulation is particularly useful when treating seborrheic dermatitis in a person with Parkinson's disease (see Table 3.42).

Target of therapy of salicylic acid/sulfur topical includes:

- Seborrheic dermatitis

Side Effects

As with most medications, side effects may occur when treatment starts, when the dose is changed, or at any time; not everyone will experience side effects. Potential side effects include:

- Burning, itching, redness of affected area

Special Considerations

- Apply twice weekly for 2 weeks.
- May be used more frequently in severe cases.
- Improvement should be noticed in 1 to 2 weeks.

Table 3.42

SALICYLIC ACID/SULFUR TOPICAL (SEBULEX® SHAMPOO)
Available over the counter and consists of 2% salicylic acid and 2% sulfur

Please refer to drug reference guides for dose ranges and a complete list of drug interactions and adverse effects.

Selenium (SELSUN®)

Selenium is used topically and stops the skin from flaking. It can be purchased over the counter (see Table 3.43).

Targets of therapy of selenium include:

- Dandruff
- Seborrheic dermatitis

Side Effects

As with most medications, side effects may occur when treatment starts, when the dose is changed, or at any time; not everyone will experience side effects. Potential side effects include:

- Skin irritation
- Hair loss
- Discoloration of hair

Special Considerations

- Selenium shampoo should be applied twice weekly for 2 weeks, but it can be used every day for severe dandruff.

Table 3.43

SELENIUM (SELSUN®)
Available as a 1% shampoo and also a 1% and 2.5% lotion

- 1–2 teaspoons should be massaged into the scalp. Leave on for 2–3 minutes. Rinse scalp completely clean.
- It is not recommended that this shampoo be used if any open type of lesion or discharge is present as it could lead to increased absorption of the product.

Please refer to drug reference guides for dose ranges and a complete list of drug interactions and adverse effects.

Tacrolimus (PROTOPIC®)

Tacrolimus is a calcineurin inhibitor (see Table 3.44). It inhibits key molecules that predispose an allergic reaction. This agent is used to treat psoriasis. The oral or systemic formulations are mostly used following organ transplant. The ointment formulation is indicated for atopic dermatitis.

Targets of therapy of topical tacrolimus include:

- Psoriasis
- Atopic dermatitis

Side Effects

As with most medications, side effects may occur when treatment starts, when the dose is changed, or at any time; not everyone will experience side effects. Potential side effects include:

- Alopecia
- Localized skin reactions (redness, itching, burning)
- Constipation
- Diarrhea

Table 3.44

TACROLIMUS (PROTOPIC®)	
Available as:	5 mg/mL IV solution (not for treatment of dermatitis) 0.5 mg, 1 mg, and 5 mg capsule (not for treatment of dermatitis) 0.03% and 0.1% ointment

- Nausea
- Vomiting
- Anemia
- Leukocytosis
- Thrombocytopenia
- Headache
- Insomnia
- Tremor
- High blood pressure
- Diabetes mellitus
- QT prolongation
- Cardiomegaly
- Hyperglycemia
- Hyperkalemia
- Hypomagnesia
- Nephrotoxicity
- Infectious disease
- Malignant lymphoma

Special Considerations

- For treatment of atopic dermatitis, apply a thin layer of ointment topically twice daily to the affected area. Rub it in gently and do not cover the area with dressings.
- Long-term use of tacrolimus is not recommended based on case reports of malignancy.
- Tacrolimus is excreted in breast milk and should be avoided in nursing mothers.
- If symptoms get worse or an infection develops, the health care provider should be contacted.
- While using this drug, exposure to natural or artificial sunlight should be minimized.
- Potential drug interactions include ziprasidone, aceclofenac, amikacin, live vaccines, caspofungin, cisplatin, cyclosporine, diclofenac, nabumetone, naproxen, neomycin, phenytoin, piroxicam, rifabutin, sirolimus, spironolactone, tobramycin, tolmetin, and triamterene.

Please refer to drug reference guides for dose ranges and a complete list of drug interactions and adverse effects.

AGENTS USED FOR URINARY PROBLEMS ASSOCIATED WITH PARKINSON'S DISEASE

Oxybutynin (OXYTROL®, DITROPAN®, DITROPAN XL®)

Oxybutynin is classified as an antimuscarinic agent (see Table 3.45). It inhibits the actions of acetycholine on the smooth muscle of the bladder. This agent relaxes the bladder, thereby decreasing the contractions that cause the urgency and frequency of urination.

Targets of therapy of oxybutynin include:

- Urinary urgency
- Urinary frequency
- Urge incontinence
- Nocturia

Side Effects

As with most medications, side effects may occur when treatment starts, when the dose is changed, or at any time; not everyone will experience side effects. Potential side effects include:

- Blurred vision
- Dry mouth
- Dry eyes
- Urinary retention
- Increased postvoid residuals
- Urinary tract infection

Table 3.45

OXYBUTYNIN (OXYTROL®)	
Ditropan® Available as: 5 mg tablets 5 mg/5 mL syrup 3.9 mg/day transdermal patch	**Ditropan XL®** Available as: 5 mg, 10 mg, and 15 mg extended release tablets. Do not chew, crush, or cut the tablet.

- Confusion and memory impairment
- Constipation
- Nausea
- Dyspepsia
- Diarrhea
- Dizziness
- Somnolence
- Abdominal pain
- Headache

Special Considerations

- Avoid use in patients with narrow-angle glaucoma, urinary retention, gastric retention, or renal disease.

Please refer to drug reference guides for dose ranges and a complete list of drug interactions and adverse effects.

Tolterodine (DETROL®, DETROL LA®)

Tolterodine is classified as an antimuscarinic agent (see Table 3.46). It works on muscarinic receptors by blocking them from the effects of acetylcholine.

Targets of therapy of tolterodine include:

- Urinary urgency
- Urinary frequency
- Urge incontinence
- Nocturia

Table 3.46

TOLTERODINE	
Detrol® Available as: 1 mg and 2 mg tablets	**Detrol LA®** Available as: 2 mg and 4 mg extended release tablets. Do not chew, crush, or cut the tablet.

Side Effects

As with most medications, side effects may occur when treatment starts, when the dose is changed, or at any time; not everyone will experience side effects. Potential side effects include:

- Dry mouth
- Dizziness
- Abdominal pain
- Constipation
- Nausea
- Headache
- Blurred vision
- Dry eyes
- Urinary retention
- Drowsiness
- Confusion

Special Considerations

- Avoid use in patients with narrow-angle glaucoma, urinary retention, gastric retention, or renal disease.

Please refer to drug reference guides for dose ranges and a complete list of drug interactions and adverse effects.

Solifenacin (VESICARE®)

Solifenacin, one of the newest muscarinic receptor antagonists, has demonstrated good efficacy and tolerability in treating urinary incontinence caused by overactive bladder syndrome (see Table 3.47). Its efficacy specific to Parkinson's disease has not been fully explored.

Table 3.47

SOLIFENACIN (VESICARE®)
Available as: 5 mg and 10 mg tablets

Targets of therapy of solifenacin include:

- Urinary urgency
- Urinary frequency
- Urge incontinence
- Nocturia

Side Effects

As with most medications, side effects may occur when treatment starts, when the dose is changed, or at any time; not everyone will experience side effects. Potential side effects include:

- Dry mouth
- Constipation
- Blurred vision
- Dry eyes
- Dizziness
- Urinary tract infection
- Urinary retention
- Confusion

Special Considerations

- Avoid use in patients with narrow-angle glaucoma, urinary retention, gastric retention, or renal disease.

Please refer to drug reference guides for dose ranges and a complete list of drug interactions and adverse effects.

Darifenacin (ENABLEX®)

Darifenacin is a potent muscarinic receptor antagonist that is marketed as the extended-release tablet Enablex®. (See Table 3.48.)

Targets of therapy of darifenacin include:

- Urinary urgency
- Urinary frequency
- Urge incontinence
- Nocturia

Table 3.48

DARIFENACIN (ENABLEX®)
Available as: 7.5 mg and 15 mg extended release tablet. Do not chew, crush, or cut the tablet.

Side Effects

As with most medications, side effects may occur when treatment starts, when the dose is changed, or at any time; not everyone will experience side effects. Potential side effects include:

- Dry mouth
- Constipation
- Dyspepsia
- Abdominal pain
- Nausea
- Diarrhea
- Urinary tract infection
- Dry eyes
- Urinary retention

Special Considerations

- Avoid use in patients with narrow-angle glaucoma, urinary retention, gastric retention, renal or hepatic disease.

Please refer to drug reference guides for dose ranges and a complete list of drug interactions and adverse effects.

AGENTS USED FOR ERECTILE DYSFUNCTION

Erectile failure is a result of the autonomic dysfunction of the process necessary for an erection to occur that is seen in individuals with Parkinson's disease. In order to improve the patient's quality of life, the physician may prescribe an agent to aid erection.

Table 3.49

SILDENAFIL (VIAGRA®)
Available as: 25 mg, 50 mg, and 100 mg tablets

Sildenafil (VIAGRA®)

Targets of therapy of sildenafil (see Table 3.49) include:

- Erectile dysfunction

Side Effects

As with most medications, side effects may occur when treatment starts, when the dose is changed, or at any time; not everyone will experience side effects. Potential side effects include:

- Atrial fibrillation
- Cardiomyopathy
- Hypotension
- Myocardial infarction
- Thromboembolic disorder
- Ventricular arrhythmia
- Flushing
- Dizziness
- Headache
- Seizure
- Vision changes, including permanent visual loss
- Priapism

Special Considerations

- Taking this agent with food can decrease the amount of drug available for the body to use; therefore, this agent will work best if taken without food.
- Do not take more than 1 tablet in 24 hours.
- Onset of action occurs in 30–60 minutes, but effects can last for 24 hours or more.

- Sexual activity is not recommended in certain cardiac conditions.
- *This class of drugs should not be used when taking **nitrates** for angina and other cardiac conditions.*
- If erection lasts for longer than 4 hours, immediate help should be sought.
- Caution should be exercised when standing up directly after sexual intercourse, as the medication can lower blood pressure and may cause fainting.

Please refer to drug reference guides for dose ranges and a complete list of drug interactions and adverse effects.

Tadalafil (CIALIS®)

Targets of therapy of tadalafil (see Table 3.50) include:

- Erectile dysfunction

Side Effects

As with most medications, side effects may occur when treatment starts, when the dose is changed, or at any time; not everyone will experience side effects. Potential side effects include:

- Chest pain
- Blood pressure changes
- Increased heart rate
- Flushing
- Dyspepsia
- Nausea
- Dry mouth

Table 3.50

TADALAFIL (CIALIS®)
Available as: 5 mg, 10 mg, and 20 mg tablets

- Diarrhea
- Muscle aches
- Back/neck pain
- Vision changes, which could include permanent visual loss

Special Considerations

- Do not take more than 1 tablet in 24 hours.
- Onset of action occurs in 20–60 minutes, and may remain effective for up to 36 hours.
- Sexual activity is not recommended in certain cardiac conditions.
- *This class of drugs should not be used when taking **nitrates** for angina and other cardiac conditions.*
- If erection lasts for longer than 4 hours, immediate help should be sought.
- Caution should be exercised when standing up directly after sexual intercourse as the medication can lower blood pressure and may cause fainting.

Please refer to drug reference guides for dose ranges and a complete list of drug interactions and adverse effects.

Vardenafil (LEVITRA®)

Targets of therapy of vardenafil (see Table 3.51) include:

- Erectile dysfunction

Side Effects

As with most medications, side effects may occur when treatment starts, when the dose is changed, or at any time; not everyone will experience side effects. Potential side effects include:

- Hypotension
- Flushing
- Dyspepsia
- Nausea
- Hepatotoxicity
- Headache

Table 3.51

VARDENAFIL (LEVITRA®)
Available as: 2.5, 5, 10, and 20 mg tablets

- Dizziness
- Visual changes, which in rare cases could include permanent visual loss

Special Considerations

- Taking this agent with food can decrease the amount of drug available for the body to use; therefore, this agent will work best if taken without food.
- Do not take more than 1 tablet in 24 hours.
- Onset of action occurs in 30–60 minutes.
- Sexual activity is not recommended in certain cardiac conditions.
- *This class of drugs should not be used when taking* ***nitrates*** *for angina and other cardiac conditions.*
- If erection lasts for longer than 4 hours, immediate help should be sought.
- Caution should be exercised when standing up directly after sexual intercourse as the medication can lower blood pressure and may cause fainting.

Please refer to drug reference guides for dose ranges and a complete list of drug interactions and adverse effects.

AGENTS USED FOR DRY EYES IN PARKINSON'S DISEASE

Hydroxypropyl Methylcellulose (NATURE'S TEARS®)

Dry eyes resulting from a decreased eye blink, normal aging, and some Parkinson medications (primarily the anticholinergic medications), can be treated with an over-the-counter eye solution such as hydroxypropyl methylcellulose (see Table 3.52). This product directly lubricates and creates a moist environment for the eyes.

Table 3.52

HYDROXYPROPYL METHYLCELLULOSE (NATURE'S TEARS®)
Available as eye drop solution or eye mist

Targets of therapy of hydroxypropyl methylcellulose include:

- Dry, itchy, red, sore eyes

Side Effects

As with most medications, side effects may occur when treatment starts, when the dose is changed, or at any time; not everyone will experience side effects. Potential side effects include:

- Rare blurred vision
- Eyelash matting

Special Considerations

- Instruct patient to wash hands prior to use.
- Do not touch tip of bottle to decrease risk of infection.
- Administer 1–2 drops into affected eye(s) as needed.
- Remove contact lenses prior to use.

Please refer to drug reference guides for dose ranges and a complete list of drug interactions and adverse effects.

AGENTS USED TO IMPROVE SLEEP/ALERTNESS IN PARKINSON'S DISEASE

Parkinson's disease and anti-Parkinson medication can sometimes make it difficult for patients to sleep. If sleep is a problem, PD medications and nonpharmacological approaches such as practicing good sleep hygiene should be optimized. In addition, some patients will need a medication to help them get a good night's sleep. Fortunately there are many medications available to help with sleep, but it may take some time and patience to find the appropriate agent for a particular patient.

Drugs have been developed to target the enzymes that are responsible for regulating the sleep/wake cycle. Currently there are four agents to choose from that are specifically marketed to facilitate sleep. They are similar in side effects, but people may respond differently to different agents. What works well for one patient may not work well for another and vice versa.

In general these agents work fairly fast to induce sleep, so it is advisable to take these medications while getting into the bed at night. It is important to know that sometimes these medications can cause drowsiness that persists into the next day and can resemble a hangover. Also, some patients feel they are much slower during the day.

Zolpidem (AMBIEN®), Zolpidem Controlled Release (AMBIEN CR®)

Zolpidem binds selectively to the benzodiazepine-1 receptor (see Table 3.53).

Targets of therapy of zolpidem include:

- Insomnia

Side Effects

As with most medications, side effects may occur when treatment starts, when the dose is changed, or at any time; not everyone will experience side effects. Potential side effects include:

- Diarrhea
- Nausea

Table 3.53

ZOLPIDEM	
Zolpidem (Ambien®)	**Zolpidem controlled release (AmbienCR®)**
Available as 5 mg and 10 mg tablets	Available as 6.25 mg and 12.5 mg tablets

- Muscle aches
- Dizziness
- Drugged state
- Headache
- Somnolence
- Depression
- Suicidal ideation
- Memory impairment
- Sleepwalking
- Increased risk of falls

Special Considerations

- Elderly patients should be monitored for excessive drowsiness and the possibility of psychomotor retardation. Changes in cognition may also occur.
- Sleepwalking episodes have been reported in some patients using zolpidem. Therefore, it is best to take this drug while getting into bed for the evening.
- It is not recommended that zolpidem be taken with alcohol because of increased cognitive and psychomotor slowing. Alcohol impairs performance and when used in conjunction with hypnotics there is an increased risk of impaired performance and reduced cognition.
- Food may decrease the amount of zolpidem that is absorbed.

Please refer to drug reference guides for dose ranges and a complete list of drug interactions and adverse effects.

Eszopiclone (LUNESTA®)

Eszopiclone interacts at the GABA receptors in the brain (see Table 3.54).

Table 3.54

ESZOPICLONE (LUNESTA®)
Available at: 1 mg, 2 mg, and 3 mg

Targets of therapy of eszopiclone include:

- Insomnia

Side Effects

As with most medications, side effects may occur when treatment starts, when the dose is changed, or at any time; not everyone will experience side effects. Potential side effects include:

- Gynecomastia
- Dyspepsia
- Nausea
- Vomiting
- Anxiety
- Depression
- Hallucinations
- Bitter taste
- Nervousness
- Decreased libido
- Somnolence
- Chest pain
- Peripheral edema

Special Considerations

- It is not recommended that eszopiclone be taken with alcohol because of increased cognitive and psychomotor slowing. Alcohol impairs performance and when used in conjunction with hypnotics there is an increased risk of impaired performance and reduced cognition.

Table 3.55

ZALEPLON (SONATA®)
Available as: 5 mg and 10 mg capsules

- Elderly patients should be monitored for excessive drowsiness and the possibility of psychomotor retardation. Changes in cognition may also occur.
- The effects may be delayed when taken with meals.

Please refer to drug reference guides for dose ranges and a complete list of drug interactions and adverse effects.

Zaleplon (SONATA®)

Zaleplon potentiates GABA (see Table 3.55).

Targets of therapy of zaleplon include:

- Insomnia

Side Effects

As with most medications, side effects may occur when treatment starts, when the dose is changed, or at any time; not everyone will experience side effects. Potential side effects include:

- Dizziness
- Somnolence
- Abdominal pain
- Headache
- Incoordination

Special Considerations

- It is not recommended that zaleplon be taken with alcohol because it may cause increased cognitive and psychomotor slowing. Alcohol impairs performance and when used in conjunction with hypnotics there is an increased risk of impaired performance and reduced cognition.
- Elderly patients should be monitored for excessive drowsiness and the possibility of psychomotor retardation. Changes in cognition may also occur.
- It is not recommended that zaleplon be taken immediately after a high-fat meal.

Please refer to drug reference guides for dose ranges and a complete list of drug interactions and adverse effects.

Ramelteon (ROZEREM®)

Ramelteon is a melatonin receptor agonist (see Table 3.56).

Targets of therapy of ramelteon include:

- Insomnia

Side Effects

As with most medications, side effects may occur when treatment starts, when the dose is changed, or at any time; not everyone will experience side effects. Potential side effects include:

- Nausea
- Dizziness
- Fatigue
- Somnolence
- Depression

Special Considerations

- It is not recommended that ramelteon be taken with alcohol because it may cause increased cognitive and psychomotor slowing. Alcohol impairs performance and when used in conjunction with hypnotics there is an increased risk of impaired performance and reduced cognition.
- Elderly patients should be monitored for excessive drowsiness and the possibility of psychomotor retardation. Changes in cognition may also occur.

Table 3.56

RAMELTEON (ROZEREM®)
Available as: an 8 mg tablet

- It is not recommended that ramelteon be taken with food or immediately after a high-fat meal because ramelteon's effects may be delayed.

Please refer to drug reference guides for dose ranges and a complete list of drug interactions and adverse effects.

Trazodone (DESYREL®)

Trazodone is primarily used for insomnia; particularly it is helpful to help individuals fall asleep as well as to lessen the occurrence of early morning awakenings. Trazodone is classified as a serotonin-adrenergic reuptake inhibitor. The agent has weak agonist/antagonist properties on serotonin receptors. It also mildly blocks adrenergic receptors. It has mild antidepressant properties, but often requires much higher doses to achieve this effect. Therefore, it is usually not the first-line choice for treatment of depression as SSRIs are now available.

Side Effects

As with most medications, side effects may occur when treatment starts, when the dose is changed, or at any time; not everyone will experience side effects. Potential side effects include:

- Changes in blood pressure
- Dizziness
- Confusion
- Drowsiness
- Headache
- Uncoordination
- Tremors
- Dry mouth
- Blurred vision
- Weight gain
- Urinary retention
- Priapism (prolonged and painful erection)

Special Considerations

- This medication should be taken with food to decrease dizziness and orthostatic hypotension.

- It is not advisable to take trazodone with alcohol because of the increased risks of central nervous system side effects and sedation.
- Patients should avoid activities that require alertness and good coordination until the CNS effects of the drug are known.
- The prescribing doctor may want to consider more conservative dosing in the elderly because trazodone can be very sedating (see Table 3.24).

Please refer to drug reference guides for dose ranges and a complete list of drug interactions and adverse effects.

Tricyclic Antidepressants (TCA)

Examples include:

Amitriptyline (ELAVIL®)

Imipramine (TOFRANIL®)

Doxepin (SINEQUAN®)

TCAs may be beneficial in patients with insomnia, bladder hyperactivity, and drooling, because of their anticholinergic effects (see Tables 3.25 and 3.26). In contrast, these anticholinergic properties may worsen cognitive impairment, hallucinations, hypotension, or excessive daytime somnolence. Depressed patients with comorbid anxiety may also respond better to SSRIs.

Side Effects

TCAs have common side effects, which include:

- Dry mouth
- Drowsiness
- Constipation
- Blurred vision
- Urinary hesitancy; incontinence
- Memory loss and cognitive slowing
- Confusion
- Hypotension; orthostasis; fainting
- Heart rhythm problems

- Sexual problems
- Weight gain

Special Considerations

- Caution must be used when prescribing this class of agents with MAO inhibitors such as rasagiline.
- This class of drugs is best avoided in the elderly, especially those with cognitive impairment, heart rhythm problems, and prostate enlargement.
- They are best used at night because of their strong sedative effects.
- It is best to start at very low doses and increase slowly for better tolerability.
- These drugs should also be avoided in patients with glaucoma or increased intraocular pressure.

Modafinil (PROVIGIL®)

Modafinil is a *nonamphetamine* stimulant (see Table 3.57). The exact mechanism of modafinil is unclear. Some reports suggest modafinil reduces levels of the neurotransmitter GABA while increasing glutamate. It may also affect histamine release. Modafinil is used in Parkinson's disease to increase alertness in individuals who report excessive daytime sleepiness.

It is not as potent as other stimulating agents including methylphenidate and amphetamines, but mood and attention improvements still occur.

There have been reports that it may also improve fatigue in Parkinson's disease, although this remains to be proven in a properly designed clinical trial.

Targets of therapy of modafinil include:

- Excessive sleepiness associated with narcolepsy, obstructive sleep apnea/hypopnea syndrome, and shift-work sleep disorder

Table 3.57

MODAFINIL (PROVIGIL®)
Available as: 100 and 200 mg tablets

- Daytime sleepiness (off-label use in Parkinson's disease)

Side Effects

As with most medications, side effects may occur when treatment starts, when the dose is changed, or at any time; not everyone will experience side effects. Potential side effects include:

- Headache
- Nausea
- Depression
- Nervousness
- Tremor
- Changes in heart rate
- Mental status changes
- Anxiety
- Insomnia
- Cataplexy
- Dyskinesia
- Diarrhea
- Dry mouth
- Increased salivation
- Anorexia

Special Considerations

- Use cautiously in patients with renal or hepatic impairment and in patients with cardiovascular disease or hypertension.

Please refer to drug reference guides for dose ranges and a complete list of drug interactions and adverse effects.

AGENTS USED TO IMPROVE BLOOD PRESSURE IN PARKINSON'S DISEASE

Fludrocortisone (FLORINEF®)

Fludrocortisone is used to treat low blood pressure, which can become pronounced upon sitting up or standing (orthostatic hypotension). (See

Table 3.58

FLUDROCORTISONE (FLORINEF®)
Available as 0.1 mg tablet

Table 3.58.) Significant drops in blood pressure may be caused by the disease itself or may be a side effect of anti-Parkinson medication.

Fludrocortisone is a corticosteroid that increases sodium reabsorption and potassium and hydrogen secretion. It helps maintain blood pressure by increasing fluid retention.

Before beginning treatment with fludrocortisone, there are some strategies to help alleviate symptoms:

- Review medication list and remove any unnecessary drugs that lower blood pressure.
- Increase salt in diet.
- Increase fluid intake (6–8 tall glasses daily).
- Elevate head of bed—raise head of bed 4–6 inches.
- Use salt tablets—1 tablet 2–3 times daily.
- Use thigh-high (tight) stockings during the day.

If orthostatic hypotension (i.e., blood pressure drops as the patient sits or stands up) is still present, then fludrocortisone may be prescribed.

Side Effects

As with most medications, side effects may occur when treatment starts, when the dose is changed, or at any time; not everyone will experience side effects. Potential side effects include:

- Hypertension
- Peripheral edema
- Hypokalemia
- Bruising
- Diaphoresis
- Urticaria

- Allergic rash
- Cardiac hypertrophy
- Heart failure

Special Considerations

- Monitor patient's blood pressure and heart rate regularly. Supine hypertension, which may occur in the evening with use of fludrocortisone, may prompt a dose reduction or use of a small dose of a blood-pressure-lowering agent only at night to address this if the pressure becomes too high.
- Monitor electrolytes on account of the risk of hypokalemia.
- Use cautiously with potassium-depleting drugs, including diuretics.
- The patient's diet should be high in potassium, with potassium supplements as needed.
- Have the patient obtain a daily weight reading and notify the health care provider of any sudden weight gain.
- Drug interactions may occur with bronchodilators, diuretics, laxatives, digitalis, barbiturates, and other corticosteroids.

Please refer to drug reference guides for dose ranges and a complete list of drug interactions and adverse effects.

Midodrine (PROAMATINE®)

Midodrine is in a class of agents known as *vasopressors* (see Table 3.59). Midodrine increases blood pressure through its action on receptors in the body that can increase blood pressure (alpha-1 receptors). Because it may increase the risk of supine hypertension, it should be avoided at night and used in carefully selected patients who have failed other attempts to maintain an adequate blood pressure. Before beginning

Table 3.59

MIDODRINE (PROAMATINE®)
Available as 2.5 mg, 5 mg, 10 mg

treatment with midodrine, there are some strategies to help alleviate symptoms:

- Review medication list and remove any unnecessary drugs that lower blood pressure.
- Increase salt in diet.
- Increase fluid intake (6–8 tall glasses daily).
- Elevate head of bed—raise head of bed 4–6 inches.
- Use salt tablets—1 tablet 2–3 time daily.
- Use thigh-high (tight) stockings during the day.

If orthostatic hypotension (i.e., blood pressure drops as the patient sits or stands up) is still present, then midodrine may be prescribed.

Targets of therapy of midodrine include:

- Orthostatic hypotension
- Hepatorenal syndrome

Side Effects

As with most medications, side effects may occur when treatment starts, when the dose is changed, or at any time; not everyone will experience side effects. Potential side effects include:

- Paresthesia
- Pruritus
- Piloerection
- Supine hypertension
- Dysuria
- Urinary retention
- Headache
- Confusion
- Dry mouth
- Anxiety

Special Considerations

- Monitor blood pressure and heart rate regularly. Supine hypertension, which may occur in the evening with use of proamatine, may prompt a dose reduction or use of a small dose of a blood-pressure-lowering agent only at night to address this if the pressure becomes too high.

- Give midodrine during the day when the patient is up and out of bed to minimize supine hypertension.
- Provide patient and family education on signs and symptoms of supine hypertension.
- Medication doses should be administered at no less than 3-hour intervals.
- Use cautiously with medications that will increase blood pressure.

Please refer to drug reference guides for dose ranges and a complete list of drug interactions and adverse effects.

Table 3.60

MEDICATIONS THAT BLOCK OR DECREASE DOPAMINE AND CAN WORSEN PARKINSON SYMPTOMS

Antipsychotic Medications	Haloperidol (Haldol® Loxapine (Loxitane®) Molindone ((Moban®) Thiothixene (Navane®) Chlorpromazine (Thorazine®) Fluphenazine (Prolixin®) Perphenazine (Trilafon®) Trifluoperazine (Stelazine®) Thioridazine (Mellaril®) Risperidone (Risperdal®) Ziprasidone (Geodon®) Olanzapine (Zyprexa®) Aripiprazole (Abilify®)
Antidepressants	Amoxapine (Ascendin®) Perphenazine/amitriptyline (Triavil®)
Antiemetics	Prochlorperazine (Compazine®) Metoclopramide (Reglan®) Thiethylperazine (Torecan®) Promethazine (Phenergan®) Droperidol (Inapsine®)
Antihypertensives	Reserpine (Serpasil®) Rauwolfia Serpentina (Raudixin®) Alpha-methyldopa (Aldomet®)

PHARMACOLOGIC AGENTS THAT SHOULD BE USED CAREFULLY OR AVOIDED IN PARKINSON'S DISEASE MANAGEMENT

Health care providers, individuals with Parkinson's disease, and family caregivers should be aware of potential drug interactions or medications that may worsen Parkinson symptoms. Fortunately most medications can be used with anti-Parkinson agents, but some drugs should not be used at all or must be used cautiously. This section will list medications that block dopamine, thereby increasing Parkinson symptoms. In addition, there are several medications that should not be used with the drug class MAO-B inhibitors, which incur an increased risk of high blood pressure, increased heart rate, seizures, fever, or confusion (see Tables 3.60–3.62).

Additional brand names may be available for each medication. Please refer to drug reference guides for a complete list.

Table 3.61

MEDICATIONS THAT SHOULD NOT BE TAKEN IN COMBINATION WITH LEVODOPA	
Antidepressants	Phenelzine (Nardil®) Tranylcypromine (Parnate®)
Iron supplements	May decrease the absorption of levodopa so should be taken at least 2 hours before or after carbidopa/levodopa

Table 3.62

MEDICATIONS THAT SHOULD NOT BE USED WITH CERTAIN MAO-B INHIBITORS: SELEGILINE (ELDEPRYL®, ZELAPAR®) AND RASAGILINE (AZILECT®)
The narcotic meperidine (Demerol®) should not be used. Patients should be taught to notify health care providers before surgery or colonoscopy is scheduled.
The antidepressant mirtazipine (Remeron®) and St. John's Wort should be avoided.
Cough medicines containing dextromethorphan should be avoided.
Cold, allergy, and sinus medications containing pseudoephedrine (Sudafed®) and ephedrine should be avoided.

B Nonpharmacological Management

CARE SETTINGS IN PARKINSON'S DISEASE

Parkinson's disease is a chronic, progressive disorder: care for individuals with this illness exists on a continuum from diagnosis to end of life. This alphabetized section will review health care and home care settings that patients may utilize and/or need throughout the trajectory of living with Parkinson's. Common concerns related to PD are included.

Adult Day Health Programs

Adult day health programs are in existence throughout the United States to provide a supportive environment for individuals who are unable to safely and/or socially remain at home during daytime hours. These settings are designed for patients to participate in community life through a variety of programs and with individuals who share common interests and needs. Licensed health care professionals are on site to provide close supervision, medical monitoring, and medication management. Rehabilitation and other types of services may be offered in some locations.

Individuals with PD utilize adult day health programs for a variety of reasons including:

- Increased need for socialization
- Assistance with management of complex medication schedules
- Assistance with mobility due to fluctuations in motor response
- Safety monitoring due to an increased risk of falls
- Assistance with activities of daily living
- Respite for family caregivers

Patients and families need encouragement and support when deciding to enroll in *day programs*. Reasons for resisting utilization of these services are varied. First of all, the financial costs associated with this type of care are often perceived as prohibitive. Most adult day programs are private pay but others may have available scholarships, grants, and/or sliding scales. Some long-term care policies, government subsidies, and Veteran's Administration programs provide coverage for qualified participants. In addition, because many Parkinson patients commonly exhibit a lack of initiative to engage in life's activities, if given the choice, they will elect to stay home and remain sedentary. Also, family caregivers often express guilt when enrolling loved ones in out-of-home programs. These feelings are compounded by thoughts that only they can provide appropriate care. Gentle persuasion is often necessary in order for patients and families to see the potential benefits of these services. Most individuals who ultimately participate in adult programs report positive experiences and an improved quality of life.

Planning ahead and taking time to select an adult day program allows for a better transition for all involved. Ideally, a program should meet the unique needs of each PD person and provide stimulating activities and social interactions with peers. Individual treatment plans should be part of the services. And, a program should have adequate staffing in order to provide anti-Parkinson medications on time. Some specialized adult day services specific to PD do exist, but they are few and far between.

Additional information on adult day health programs can be obtained by visiting the Web site of the National Adult Day Services Association (www.nadsa.org).

Assisted Living Communities

The number of assisted living communities throughout the United States has grown significantly in recent years. This homelike setting is designed typically for seniors who are no longer able, for a wide variety of reasons, to live independently but who do not require the level of care provided in a nursing home. Services include assistance with activities of daily living and management of medications that are essential for individuals affected by PD. Most communities provide licensed nursing and rehabilitation services. Other beneficial outreach includes recreational and social programs, exercise and fitness classes, and in some circumstances, on-site PD support groups.

Useful resources about these communities for health care providers to assist patients and families include:

- The National Center for Assisted Living (www.ncal.org)
- American Assisted Living Nurses Association (www.alnursing.org)
- American Association of Homes and Services for the Aging (www.aahsa.org)
- Long-Term Care Living (www.longtermcareliving.com)
- A Place for Mom (www.aplaceformom.com)

Emergency Room Care

Individuals with Parkinson's disease most often visit an emergency room for the following reasons:

- An acute change in mental status including an increase in anxiety, confusion, hallucinations, and/or psychosis
- An acute change in medical condition such as a pneumonia, bladder infection, bowel obstruction, and so forth
- An injury related to a fall, such as a hip fracture
- A worsening of Parkinson symptoms not associated with another condition, such as an extended "off" period or an increase in dyskinesia
- Caregiver burnout and/or lack of support services in the home

The emergency room should be used for emergencies only. Emergency rooms may be inappropriately utilized when adequate communication systems are not in place for individuals to access acute medical care. This, coupled with patient and family anxiety and stress with a change in condition, increases the likelihood of using an ER. Therefore, patients and family members should be aware of how and when to access their health care providers should a change in medical condition occur.

Being prepared for an emergency medical situation will result in efficient and enhanced care when it is necessary. Patients and family/caregivers should maintain current health records, including an updated list of medications with times of administration, a list of medications to avoid, physician contacts including the Parkinson disease specialist, and other information that will be useful for the ER staff.

Home Care

Home care is provided for individuals with Parkinson's disease by primary and secondary caregivers. Primary caregivers are generally family members, usually a spouse, or close friends. Secondary caregivers include individuals who provide skilled care such as licensed nurses, physical therapists, occupational therapists, speech and language pathologists, social workers, and home health aides. Also, there are those who provide nonskilled care. These are homemakers and personal care attendants.

Home health care agencies exist to provide comprehensive home care services. They may be for-profit, nonprofit, or governmental. The programs may provide skilled services or nonskilled services or both. Skilled services may be reimbursable by insurance coverage for a certain period of time. Nonskilled services are reimbursed only by certain long-term-care insurances and private pay.

Referrals for skilled services can be made from hospital and short-term rehabilitation facility discharge planners as well as directly from a patient's physician. Certain criteria exist that must be fulfilled for a Parkinson's patient to receive reimbursable skilled home care, including having a certain period of being homebound.

Skilled home care is added if there is a change in health status, a change in functional status, or a knowledge deficit related to a change in medical treatment. One example includes the PD patient who has a change in functional status related to an increase in PD symptoms. This person may need daily assessment to determine if a new medication plan is working. Assessment may include level of function in relation to time of medication intake, cognition and mood, and ability to move safely. PD medication schedules are complex and require careful organization. Licensed nurses can assist patients with this task.

Hospitalization

Admission to a hospital presents certain challenges to the Parkinson patient and family. Health care professionals play a significant role in helping patients overcome these challenges. Reasons for hospital admissions include an acute worsening of PD symptoms, changes in mental status including onset of moderate to severe hallucinations and confusion, infection, pneumonia, other comorbidities, and injury from a fall. In addition, patients are admitted for elective procedures including deep brain stimulation as well as any other non-PD-related illnesses or procedures.

Following a hospitalization, many PD patients are transferred to acute rehabilitation or short-term nursing units for continued care. The slower-paced environment and available rehabilitation services usually decrease problems or complications associated with an acute hospital setting.

There are common issues associated with hospital admissions for PD patients:

- Very often, patients do not receive the right dosage of medication on time. This is usually the number one concern for both the patients and family caregivers. PD medication schedules are complex, requiring frequent dosing throughout the day. These medications provide symptom relief. Patients who have motor fluctuations are at the greatest risk of decreased mobility if medication schedules are altered. Patients and families should provide hospital staff with clearly outlined instructions, including names of medications, doses, and times of administration. Physicians or nurses should inform patients when medication adjustments will be made and provide reasons for the adjustment. Health care providers should be aware of medications that will increase Parkinson symptoms. A complete list of medications contraindicated in Parkinson's disease is included in the section prior to this entitled "Pharmacological Management."
- Hospital personnel, including physicians and nursing staff, are sometimes not familiar with the specialized and individualized needs of PD patients. This unfamiliarity in part results from a paucity of education and training in PD. One common misunderstanding relates to motor fluctuations. For example, personnel may not understand why a person can move well in the morning yet be totally immobile in the afternoon.
- Parkinson disease physicians caring for the admitted patient may not be associated with the hospital. Patients and family members should inform the Parkinson physician about a hospitalization as soon as it is known. It is helpful to provide the name and contact

number of the Parkinson-treating physician to the admitting hospital physician. Patients may also benefit from a consultation by the hospital neurology team.

- Many PD patients are prevented from physically communicating with personnel by the illness. Many have speech problems, including low voice volume, dysarthria, and slowness in response time. Nurses and physicians may interpret this as confusion. Communication problems should be identified and discussed at admission.
- Increased confusion or disorientation may often be seen in the hospital setting. This confusion may be a reason for admission but often will occur because patients are out of their normal environments and are in settings with unfamiliar people, sights, and sounds. Infection will also increase the risk of confusion. This potential for confusion is one of the many reasons that support discussion and completion of advance directives (durable power of attorney and a living will) by the patient and family caregiver well before any change in health status.
- Increased immobility is often seen during hospitalization. Patients who need assistance with mobility or who are unable to move are at greater risk of problems associated with immobility. Patients may have intact gross motor movements but may have difficulty with fine motor movements. For example, patients may be able to feed themselves independently but cannot get lids off of juice containers or cut food into small pieces. Health care providers should assist with activities of daily living as needed. They should also ambulate patients regularly. A referral for physical and occupational therapy should be made during admission.
- Increased risk of injury from a fall is a common concern. Safety precautions are important for Parkinson patients in any environment. A mobility and transfer plan including availability of assistive devices should be established at admission.

Proper planning and positive communication between the patient, family, and health care providers can alleviate many of the problems associated with hospitalization.

Long-Term Care

Admission to a long-term care nursing facility occurs when a person is unable to provide self-care or receive care at home. The American Medical

Director Association estimates that 5%–7% of individuals in nursing homes have Parkinson's disease, dementia with Lewy bodies, vascular parkinsonism or other parkinsonian conditions. Those with PD typically have some cognitive impairment; often qualifying for a diagnosis of PD dementia.

The already complex care needs of the PD patient increase when admitted to a nursing facility. Reasons for admission include one or more of the following: increased hallucinations, confusion, psychosis, and the inability to perform activities of daily living including dressing, toileting, feeding, and transfer in and out of bed. It is imperative to receive care that will prevent further complications. Nursing and rehabilitation staff should be familiar with the care needs of the patient. Staff education personnel should identify and support the educational needs of health care professionals in their care setting. Lay organizations including the American Parkinson Disease Association and the National Parkinson Disease Foundation have developed educational materials for patients, families, and health care staff. APDA Information and Referral Center Coordinators often arrange in-services for nurses and therapists.

Family members often have strong feelings that they have failed their loved one and require significant support around this placement decision. In most cases they have worked tirelessly caring for the person with PD. They should have a significant role in developing the nursing care plan.

Resources for Health Care Professionals

American Medical Directors Association. (2002). *Parkinson's disease in the long-term care setting: Guidelines and an algorithm of care for health care professionals.* Columbia, MD: Author. Print copies: Available from the American Medical Directors Association, 10480 Little Patuxent Pkwy., Suite 760, Columbia, MD 21044. Telephone: 800-876-2632 or 410-740-9743; fax 410-740-4572. Web site: www.amda.com.

To Share With Families

Bornstein, R. F., & Languirand, M. A. (2001). *When someone you love needs nursing home care: The complete guide.* New York: Newmarket Press.

Movement Disorder Centers

Movement Disorder Centers provide highly specialized and comprehensive care to individuals and families affected by Parkinson's disease or other movement disorders. These centers also participate in the latest research and provide specialized training to medical students, residents, fellows, and other health care providers. In addition, patients, family members, and the community at large benefit from educational and support programs of the center designed to increase an understanding of the disease process, bolster self-efficacy, and improve quality of life.

Many centers have a multidisciplinary care model with health care providers from more than one discipline. All centers have a movement disorder specialist who is a neurologist who has had significant experience and training in movement disorders. Depending on the scope of care provided at a center, team members may include movement disorder nurses, nurse practitioners, physician assistants, rehabilitation specialists, social workers, neuropsychologists, and research coordinators.

There are different ways to locate a movement disorder neurologist and/or a movement disorder center.

- Most specialists are members of the Movement Disorder Society. The MDS does not provide a list of membership to the public, but they do have a Web site that provides information on this specialty (www.movementdisorders.org).
- Parkinson lay organizations do provide information based on specialty and location. They will not endorse one specialist over another. For additional information:
  - American Parkinson Disease Association (www.apdaparkinson.org), 800-223-2732. The Web site lists contact information for local information and referral centers.
  - National Parkinson Foundation (www.parkinson.org) or 800-327-4545. The Web site has a movement disorder specialist locator as well as an "Ask the Doctor" online discussion board.
  - Parkinson Disease Foundation (www.pdf.org) or 800-457-6676. This Web site includes information on movement disorder centers and specialists.
  - We Move (www.wemove.org). This Web site includes a movement disorder specialist locator.
  - Local Parkinson support group members will often provide information on Parkinson doctors in the area.

Palliative/End-of-Life Care

Parkinson's disease is a chronic progressive condition that individuals will have until the end of their lives. Significant advances in treatments have greatly improved life expectancy, but as with all humans, the Parkinson patient's life will come to an end. Some individuals will not advance beyond the middle stages of the disease; others will advance to late-stage disease before death. Disease progression significantly impacts the care and support that a patient and family will require at the end of life.

Health care professionals must be prepared and willing to offer treatment, guidance, and emotional support to the patient and family as the patient nears the end of life. The patient and family will benefit from supportive discussion and good information to help plan for the future, no matter how long the patient's life will be. This may include information on advanced directives, living wills, and power of attorney. Treatment options and where care will be provided should be clearly outlined. Some patients will remain at home and some will receive care in a nursing facility. Hospice services can be utilized in most settings. Discussions on end of life are often difficult. In many situations long-term relationships have been established between the patient and health care provider. Disciplines including nursing, social work, pastoral care, and hospice are available to provide physical, emotional, and spiritual care to the patient and family.

Resources

Caring Connections (National Hospice and Palliative Care Organization), www.caringinfo.org, 800-658-8898.

National Institute of Aging. (2008). *End of life: Helping with comfort and care.* Bethesda, MD: National Institute of Aging. This 72-page booklet contains information useful to patients, families, and health care professionals (www.nia.nih.gov).

COMPLEMENTARY THERAPIES

For years PD patients have used and reported efficacy with certain complimentary and alternative therapies, particularly those that improve movement and promote relaxation (e.g., meditation, tai chi, yoga.) The National Center for Complementary and Alternative Medicine (CAM), a branch of the National Institutes of Health, defines this discipline as a group of diverse medical and health care systems, practices, and products that are not presently considered to be part of conventional medicine. CAM encompasses many types of therapies including but not limited to:

- Mind-body medicine (meditation, music, and dance therapy)
- Biologically based medicine (vitamins, herbs)
- Manipulative and body-based practices (reflexology, massage)
- Energy medicine (Reiki, Qigong)
- Whole medicine systems (homeopathic medicine, ayurveda)

During the past decade there has been increased interest in studying the relationship of some of these therapies with PD. Small studies have been done evaluating tai chi, Pilates, acupuncture, and Qigong, to name a few. Some large federally funded studies are now under way. Evidence-based practice is always desired. However, study limitations include a lack of funding to conduct these studies as well as difficulty measuring efficacy, a problem that exists when studying alternative therapies.

Patients are interested in these practices. Health care professionals should become familiar with complementary and alternative therapy and be willing to provide an opinion on their use. The National Center for Complementary and Alternative Medicine provides an extensive updated Web site at www.nccam.nih.gov.

The Office of Dietary Supplements cautions that published analyses of herbal supplements have found differences between ingredients listed on the label and actual ingredients. The word *standardized* on a product label is not a guarantee of higher product quality, since in the United States there is no legal definition of *standardized* for supplements.

The following are examples of alternative therapies that have been used in PD:

Acupuncture

- Acupuncture has been practiced for over 3,000 years. Its biological mechanism of action is poorly defined. It is usually not covered by insurance and requires multiple treatments.
- Most reported studies of acupuncture are open label. In one study that examined the safety and efficacy of acupuncture in 20 patients with Parkinson's disease, while 85% of the patients reported subjective improvement of symptoms, the qualitative measures did not show significant improvement except in the areas of sleep and rest.
- Therefore, scientific evidence is still insufficient to routinely recommend the use of acupuncture to treat Parkinson's disease.

Chelation Therapy

- Chelation therapy removes heavy metals from the body.
- It is not a procedure without significant side effects and there is no scientific evidence to support its use in PD.

Coenzyme Q10 (CoQ10)

- Coenzyme Q10 is an antioxidant that is currently being investigated as a neuroprotective agent in PD and other neurodegenerative disorders.
- A well-designed preliminary study in PD found that patients placed on 1,200 mg of coenzyme Q10 daily had a reduced rate of deterioration in motor function over a 16-month period. A larger, more definitive study is currently under way to confirm this earlier finding.
- In the meantime, coenzyme Q10 is usually not covered by insurance and the high doses are relatively expensive.

Curcumin (Turmeric)

- Curcumin is an antioxidant derived from the curry spice turmeric.
- There are no data available for treatment of PD.

DHEA (Dehydroepiandrosterone)

- DHEA is an endogenous hormone.
- DHEA can cause higher than normal levels of estrogen in the body, which may modulate brain neurotransmitters and potentially have neuroprotective effects.
- This remains to be proven in PD.

Glutathione

- Glutathione is an antioxidant that is not covered by insurance and is relatively expensive.
- It has been given orally and also intravenously.
- While there have been several anecdotal and open-label reports of this drug in PD, well-designed, blinded, and placebo-controlled trials have yet to be reported at the time of this writing.

Massage Therapy

- Massage therapy consists of gentle stroking and kneading of muscles as well as other soft tissue and manual deep-tissue techniques.
- Types of massage include aromatherapy, craniofacial, lymphatic, myofascial, reflexology, shiatsu, sports, Swedish, and trigger point.
- There is no solid evidence to support benefits of routine massage therapy for PD. It frequently requires multiple treatments and is often not covered by insurance.

Tai Chi

- Tai chi combines the soft and slow movement of yoga and the calmness and relaxation of meditation.
- While there are increasing reports of tai chi improving balance and walking, well-designed studies supporting the practice of tai chi in improving symptoms of PD are still to be reported.

Vitamins E and C

- Vitamins E and C are also antioxidants.
- Observational studies suggested that Vitamin E may have a neuroprotective effect on decreasing the risk of Parkinson's disease.

There have been several large studies on vitamins E and C that found that neither intake of these two vitamin supplements (or multivitamins) was significantly associated with decreased risk of PD.

EDUCATION AND SUPPORT

Individuals with Parkinson's disease and their families require ongoing education and support throughout the course of their illness. A better understanding of PD results in more effective coping and proper long-term management. Each person requires information and planning that is carefully tailored to his or her unique situation. Members of the health care team play a significant role in assessing the specific learning needs of this population. Each patient/family interaction is an opportunity to share information that is current, evidence-based, and, most importantly, useful.

This section will highlight some organizations, supportive services, and resources available to patients, families, health care professionals, and the community at large.

Lay Organizations

Several organizations exist on both the national and local level to provide education, supply support, increase awareness, and raise important funds for research. Listed below are groups that have a national focus. For complete information visit each Web site or request information by telephone.

American Parkinson Disease Association (APDA)
www.apdaparkinson.org
135 Parkinson Avenue
Staten Island, NY 10305
Phone: 800-223-2732 or 718-981-8001
Fax: 718-981-4399
E-mail: apda@apdaparkinson.org

APDA National Young Onset Center
2100 Pfingsten Road
Glenview, IL 60026
Phone: 877-223-3801
Fax: 847-657-5708
E-mail: apda@youngparkinson.org

The Michael J. Fox Foundation for Parkinson's Research
www.MichaelJFox.org
Church Street Station
P.O. Box 780
New York, NY 10008-0780
Phone: 800-708-7644

National Parkinson Foundation
www.parkinson.org
1501 N.W. 9th Avenue/Bob Hope Road
Miami, FL 33136-1494

Phone: 305-243-6666
Toll Free National: 800-327-4545
Fax: 305-243-5595
E-mail: contact@parkinson.org

Ask the Doctor-Ask the Surgeon-Ask the Nutritionist Discussion Forum
http://forum.parkinson.org/forum/

Parkinson's Disease Foundation
www.pdf.org
1359 Broadway, Suite 1509
New York, NY 10018
Phone: 800-457-6676 or 212-923-4700
Fax: 212-923-4778
E-mail: info@pdf.org

Parkinson's Action Network
www.parkinsonsaction.org
1025 Vermont Ave NW, Suite 1120
Washington, DC 20005
Phone: 202-638-4101
Toll Free: 800-850-4726
Fax: 212-638-7257
E-mail: info@parkinsonsaction.org

The Parkinson Alliance
www.parkinsonalliance.org
P.O. Box 308
Kingston, NJ 08528-0308
Phone: 800-579-8440 or 609-688-0870
Fax: 609-688-0875

WE MOVE–Worldwide Education and Awareness for Movement Disorders
www.wemove.org
204 West 84th Street
New York, NY 10024
E-mail: wemove@wemove.org

World Parkinson Disease Association
http://www.wpda.org/

World Parkinson Congress
www.worldpdcongress.org

Professional Organizations

American Academy of Neurology (AAN)
www.aan.com
1080 Montreal Avenue
Saint Paul, MN 55116
Phone: 800-879-1960 or 651-695-2717
Fax: 651-695-2791
E-mail: memberservices@aan.com

American Association of Neuroscience Nurses (AANN)
www.aann.org
4700 W. Lake Avenue
Glenview, IL 60025
Phone: 888-557-2266 (United States only)
or 847-375-4733
Fax: 847-375-6430
Int'l Fax: 732-460-7313
E-mail: info@aann.org

American Medical Directors Association (AMDA)
www.amda.com
11000 Broken Land Parkway, Suite 400
Columbia, MD 21044
Phone: 410-740-9743
Toll Free: 800-876-2632
Fax: 410-740-4572

American Physical Therapy Association (APTA)
www.apta.org
1111 North Fairfax Street
Alexandria, VA 22314-1488
Phone: 800/999-APTA (2782)
703-684-APTA (2782)
TDD: 703-638-6748
Fax: 703-684-7343

American Occupational Therapy Association (AOTA)
www.aota.org

4720 Montgomery Lane
P.O. Box 31220
Bethesda, MD 20824-1220
Phone: 301-652-2682
TDD: 800-377-8555
Fax: 301-652-7711

American Speech-Language-Hearing Association (ASHA)
www.asha.org
ASHA National Office
2200 Research Boulevard
Rockville, MD 20850-3289
Phone: 301-296-5700

Movement Disorder Society (MDS)
www.movementdisorders.org
International Secretariat
555 East Wells Street, Suite 1100
Milwaukee, WI 53202-3823 (USA)
Phone: 414-276-2145
Fax: 414-276-3349
E-mail: info@movementdisorders.org

National Association of Social Workers (NASW)
www.socialworkers.org
750 First Street, NE, Suite 700
Washington, DC 20002-4241
Phone: 202-408-8600

Support Groups

Support groups exist all over the world to help individuals with Parkinson's disease and their family members better cope with this chronic condition. Meetings that are offered, both formal and informal, accomplish this by providing education, socialization, coping strategies, and mutual support. Most groups follow a self-help model. This means they are member-run and are composed of individuals who share the same situation (a diagnosis of PD). Some groups will share facilitator duties with a health care professional, most often a social worker or nurse.

There are limited studies of the benefits of PD support groups; however, their increasing numbers and widespread participation support the importance of their existence.

Choosing when and if to join a group is an important decision for a patient and family. Each group's function is uniquely dependent on a number of factors: group location, age of the members, years in existence, and group leadership, to name a few. Just as with anything, what works for one person may not work for another, therefore, individuals may visit more than one group to find the best fit.

Specialty groups exist within the PD support-group network. For instance, there are groups for young individuals with PD (young-onset groups), caregivers, or individuals who have or are considering deep brain stimulation (DBS).

As a health care professional, it is often difficult to recommend a support group when one is not familiar with the group's dynamics. It is important to know what groups exist in a local area. It is useful to take the time to speak with the group leader and learn as much as possible about the group. In addition, group members benefit from the expertise of a health care professional and are often delighted to incorporate an educational presentation into their meeting.

To locate a list of support groups in your area contact the American Parkinson Disease Association (www.apdaparkinson.org) or the National Parkinson Foundation (www.Parkinson.org). These organizations support local centers that assist with the development and maintenance of support groups. Many groups publicize their activities in local newspapers, hospitals, and community centers.

Information on Parkinson Disease Research Studies and Clinical Trials

PD Trials—An initiative to increase education and awareness of clinical trials led by the Parkinson Disease Foundation in collaboration with other organizations.
www.pdtrials.org
E-mail: info@pdtrials.org
Phone: 800-457-6676

Parkinson Study Group (PSG)—A cooperative group of Parkinson's disease experts from medical centers in the United States and Canada

who are dedicated to improving treatment for persons affected by Parkinson's disease.
www.parkinson-study-group.org
University of Rochester
1351 Mt. Hope Ave., Suite 223
Rochester, NY 14620

National Institutes of Health
www.clinical trials.gov

National Institute of Neurological Disorders and Stroke
www.ninds.nih.gov

Parkinson's Disease Pipeline
www.pdpipeline.org

PHYSICAL THERAPY

Physical therapy is an important discipline in the management of Parkinson's disease. Results of large-scale studies have shown the benefits of physical therapy and exercise on both function and quality of life. Currently, research is ongoing to determine if exercise might have a neuroprotective effect and slow the progression of the disease. Although not conclusive, this possibility is one more reason why individuals with a diagnosis of PD should participate in a regular, well-designed exercise program.

Physical therapists are licensed health care professionals that are trained to examine an individual's physical impairments, functional status, and quality of life. Treatment includes strategies aimed at prevention, restoration, and/or compensation.

Areas of Assessment

Functional Status

- Walking
- Rising from a chair
- Bed mobility
- Balance
- Upper-extremity function

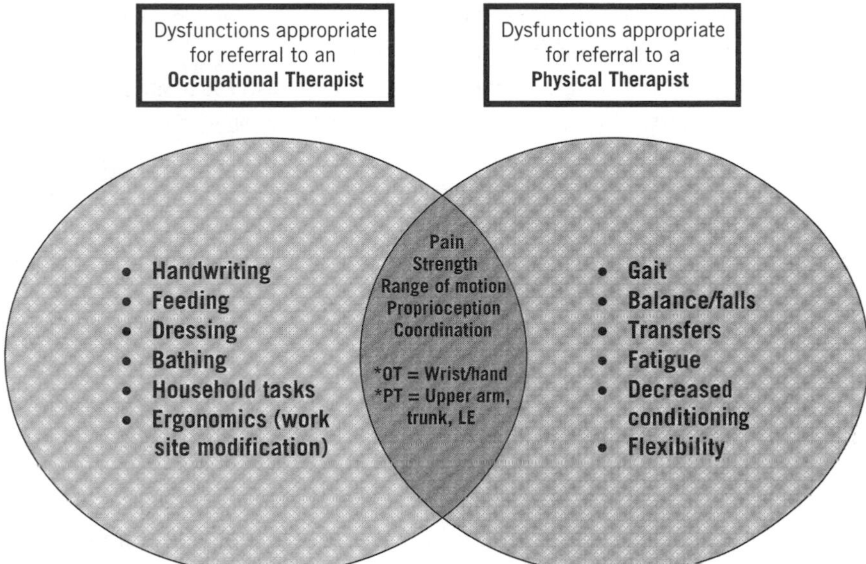

Figure 3.1 Issues addressed by physical and occupational therapists.

Physical Impairments

- Rigidity
- Bradykinesia
- Tremor
- Range of Motion
- Strength
- Coordination
- Endurance

In order for PD patients to receive the maximum benefit from therapy, it is important that the appropriate referral is made. Patients will gain the most benefit from an early referral to initiate education and prevention strategies. This includes making a referral to the right discipline in the right rehabilitation setting (see Figure 3.1).

Treatment Strategies

- Gait training to increase step length and overcome gait freezing
- Use of music or metronome with specific beats to increase speed and quality of gait

- Strategies to improve functional mobility: sit-to-stand, bed mobility
- Fall prevention and balance training
- Strengthening, range of motion, flexibility, and endurance training
- Assessment of need for assistive devices

Evidence strongly suggests that early intervention is valuable in Parkinson's disease. A well-designed treatment and exercise program incorporating gait training, strengthening, ROM, flexibility, and endurance training should be continued over the long term.

Exercise programs specific to Parkinson's disease exist in many locations throughout the United States. Individuals may also participate in local community programs (e.g., Young Men's Christian Association [YMCA]; Jewish Community Center [JCC]). A physical therapist can provide referral to these programs. Individuals often need strong encouragement to exercise and remain active. Group programs can be highly motivating and offer the added benefit of a social component.

Assistive devices are sometimes utilized to increase safety and ease with ambulation and transfers. However, not all people who have difficulty in these areas will benefit from the use of an assistive device. Physical therapists can evaluate whether an assistive device is indicated and provide the necessary education and training in its proper use.

Educational Resources for Patients Written by Physical Therapists

Cianci, H. (2006). *Parkinson's disease fitness counts* (3rd ed.). Miami, FL: National Parkinson Foundation. www.parkinson.org

Ellis, T. P., Rork T., & Dalton, D. (2008). *Be active: An exercise program for people with Parkinson's disease.* New York: American Parkinson Disease Association. www.apdaparkinson.org

PSYCHOSOCIAL SUPPORT

Providing psychosocial evaluation and treatment is an important component in the management of patients and families with PD. This care is best delivered by a mental health professional. There are many types of mental health professionals, including psychiatrists, clinical psychologists, psychotherapists, clinical social workers, psychiatric clinical nurse specialists, and psychiatric nurses. Each discipline provides care to the PD patient and family but with a different scope of practice. For example, a psychiatrist, as a physician, will use a biomedical approach in the diagnosis and management of the patient. A clinical psychologist is specially trained in psychotherapy including cognitive behavioral therapy as well as the administration of standardized tests to assess personality, intelligence, memory, and mood. A licensed social worker provides counseling and support to patients and families and also specializes in case management and advocacy.

PD problems addressed by mental health professionals include:

- Anxiety
- Depression
- Apathy
- Fatigue
- Compulsive disorders
- Psychosis
- Dementia
- Alteration in family processes
- Social isolation
- Alteration in role performance
- Self-care deficit

Interventions include:

- Diagnosis and medical management of psychiatric problems (psychiatry)
- Psychotherapy
- Neuropsychological testing
- Relaxation therapy
- Biofeedback
- Patient/family counseling
- Support group facilitation

OCCUPATIONAL THERAPY

Occupational therapy is a health care discipline that individuals with Parkinson's disease can participate in and benefit from at all stages of their condition. Occupational therapists are licensed health care professionals who focus on a person's ability to perform activities of daily living, work, socializing, and participating in leisure activities. Careful assessment of a person's motor and nonmotor signs and symptoms and living environment (home, work, and community) is done to determine the best plan of care to restore and/or maintain function.

Activities of Daily Living Addressed

- Grooming
- Meal preparation
- Eating
- Handwriting
- Computer use
- Bed mobility
- Transfer mobility
- Homemaking
- Management of finances
- Shopping
- Driving

Occupational therapists (OTs) pay particular attention to upper-body mobility, concentrating on upper-extremity range of motion, strength, and coordination. They evaluate an individual's need for assistive devices that promote independence. Recommendations are made to improve a person's ability to not only increase function but perform activities safely. OTs often work closely with other rehabilitation specialists, including physical therapists and speech and language pathologists. An occupational therapy evaluation requires an order from the patient's health care prescriber.

When to Refer to an OT

- To obtain baseline evaluations on the degree of motor disorder, active functional movement, dependence level in activities of daily living, speed of performance of self-care activities, handwriting skills, and ability to perform simultaneous and sequential tasks
- To provide instruction in accommodation principles that can be used throughout the progression of PD
- To prevent musculoskeletal deficits
- To initiate environmental adaptations

- To provide the caregiver with instruction in the disease process and the process of rehabilitation
- To provide patient and caregiver support

Examples of OT Solutions to Common PD Problems

- Poor gait rhythm: multisensory cuing, cognitive cuing strategies
- Poor motor dexterity: coordination drills
- Fatigue: energy conservation techniques
- Declining ability to perform activities of daily living
  - Self-care: Devices and techniques are provided to reduce dependence. Practice in a monitored setting with devices is necessary for devices to be incorporated into patient's activity routines.
  - Home management: Lightweight vacuum cleaners and dust mops, jar openers, long-handled scrub brushes, and other devices may be considered to facilitate independence. Home assessments may be performed to evaluate for safety hazards such as throw rugs, or for provision of adaptive devices such as handicapped bars, shower seats, ramps, or other devices designed to improve function in the home.
- Handwriting: Exercises may be given to improve hand manipulation skills and independent finger movements.

Educational Resources for Patients Written by Occupational Therapists

Cianci, H., Cloete, L., Gardner, J., Trail, M., & Wichman, R. (2006). *Activities of daily living: Practical pointers for Parkinson disease.* Miami, FL: National Parkinson Foundation.

Clapcich, J., Goldberg, N., & Walsh, E. (2008). *Be independent: A guide for people with Parkinson's disease* (rev. ed.). New York: American Parkinson Disease Association.

Occupational Therapy Professional Organization

The American Occupational Therapy Association, Inc. (AOTA)
4720 Montgomery Lane
P.O. Box 31220
Bethesda, MD 20824-1220
301-652-2682
www.aota.org

SLEEP HYGIENE

Practicing good sleep hygiene is important for the person with Parkinson's disease and the family care provider. Getting a good night's sleep is important so that a person feels rested during the next day. Sleep deprivation will affect mobility and one's overall sense of well-being. Patients who do not sleep well report increased fatigue.

Patient and family teaching includes:

- Maintain a regular sleep schedule 7 days a week. Keep the same bedtime each night. Take bedtime medications at the same time each evening.
- Make the sleep environment as comfortable as possible. Consider a bed with capability to elevate head. Use satin sheets to move more easily. Install a grab bar or mobility transfer handle to assist with turning and getting in and out of bed. Have a comfortable recliner chair in room. Keep bedroom clear of clutter.
- Avoid stimulants including caffeine, nicotine, and alcohol too close to bedtime.
- Participate in an active exercise program during the day.
- Spend part of the day outdoors, increasing natural exposure to light.
- Avoid heavy meals within 4 hours of bedtime.
- Limit fluid intake 4 hours before bedtime.

Review Parkinson and concomitant medications with health care provider to determine if they interfere with sleep. Optimize medication schedule with health care provider.

SPEECH AND LANGUAGE PATHOLOGY

A speech and language pathologist provides prevention, diagnosis, and rehabilitation of problems associated with speech, language, swallowing, and the cognitive aspects of communication. In Parkinson's disease, individuals may experience problems with hypokinetic dysarthria (difficulty speaking clearly) and dysphagia (difficulty swallowing). In addition, mild cognitive changes can impact a person's linguistic ability.

Hypokinetic dysarthria occurs in over 50% of all individuals with PD at some point in their illness. It may be the presenting symptom of neurological disease in PD. Hypokinetic dysarthria is characterized by a breathy and hoarse voice and reduced loudness. Individuals with PD appear to have a perceptual disconnect between their actual loudness level and their own internal perception of loudness (they think they are speaking normally, or loudly, when they are actually quiet). Communication partners may have a hard time hearing their speech, especially at a distance, in a noisy environment, or on the telephone. Patients may also report avoiding social situations that require speech. The severity of speech disorders may not correspond to the duration of PD or severity of other motor symptoms. *Hyperkinetic dysarthria,* rather than *hypokinetic dysarthria,* may also be encountered. This most often occurs in the presence of dyskinesias, particularly after prolonged levodopa therapy.

Oropharyngeal dysphagia is reported in up to 95% of patients with PD, depending on the method of assessment. However, dysphagia is often unrecognized or underestimated by patients. Like dysarthria, the severity of dysphagia may not correspond to the duration of PD or severity of other motor symptoms. All stages of swallowing function can be affected in patients with PD including the oral, pharyngeal, and esophageal stages.

Areas of Assessment

- Phonation
- Resonance
- Voice pitch
- Articulation
- Linguistic ability
- Swallowing ability
- Hearing
- Facial expression

Treatment

Speech and Language

- Comprehensive voice evaluation
- Hearing assessment
- Lee Silverman Voice Treatment Program (LSVT), which has literature supporting its beneficial effects and is a popular treatment choice for individuals with PD and hypokinetic dysarthria

  - LSVT emphasizes phonatory effort and uses maximum performance tasks as the basis of intervention.
  - LSVT also "recalibrates" an individual's perceived level of effort with an emphasis on self-awareness.
  - LSVT is based upon the premise that treatment should be simple and intensive.
  - Although intact cognition is a positive prognostic indicator of success, LSVT can also be beneficial for patients with cognitive deficits.
- Other treatments as appropriate include rate control techniques and the use of delayed auditory feedback
- Augmentative-alternative communication (AAC) treatment approaches that may also be beneficial, particularly as dysarthria progresses
  - Voice amplifiers may be beneficial to increase vocal loudness.
  - Pacing boards may assist in rate control.
  - Alphabet boards may be an effective strategy to supplement speech and provide context for communication partners.
  - Other AAC strategies such as communication boards/notebooks, voice output computer systems, and portable typing devices may also be used.

Swallowing

- Conduct a modified barium swallow evaluation.
- Provide strategies to improve swallowing techniques.
- Although dysphagia is common in PD, it rarely is severe enough to require an alternative means of nutritional support. However, gastrostomy may be considered for some patients as an efficient means to provide additional nutritional support. In some situations, oral intake may continue with the presence of a gastrostomy tube.

The Effect of Medications on Communication

- For most individuals with PD, pharmacological treatment does not appear to have a significant beneficial impact on speech production.
- Hyperkinetic dysarthria, often in the presence of dyskinesias after prolonged levodopa therapy, may also be encountered.

Surgical Treatments and Communication

- Surgical treatments for PD do not have consistent significant benefit for the communication impairments associated with PD.

Patient Educational Resources Prepared by Speech and Language Pathologists

Johnson, M. L. (2005). *Parkinson disease: Speech and swallowing* (2nd ed.). Miami, FL: National Parkinson Foundation.

Lee Silverman Voice Treatment (LSVT). www.lsvt.org

Ruddy, B. H., & Sapienza, C. (2003). *Speaking effectively: A strategic guide for speaking and swallowing.* New York: American Parkinson Disease Association.

Professional Organization for Speech and Language Pathologists

American Speech-Language-Hearing Association (ASHA)
www.asha.org
2200 Research Blvd.
Rockville, MD 20850-3289

SURGERY FOR PARKINSON'S DISEASE

Surgical treatments for PD include *deep brain stimulation* (DBS) and the now rarely performed ablative procedures *thalamotomy* and *pallidotomy.* DBS can be performed unilaterally or bilaterally to treat medication-resistant motor symptoms of PD.

The procedure involves implanting an electrode stereotactically placed into a target nucleus such as the globus pallidus internus (GPi), or the subthalamic nucleus (STN). The thalamus can also be a target for individuals with severe tremor. Studies are ongoing to determine whether one of these targets is more efficacious and if there are other target areas of the brain useful in PD.

The electrodes are stimulated and adjusted through connection to a pacemakerlike device located under the skin in the chest. The means by which DBS therapy works remains unknown; however, the high-frequency, pulsatile, electrical stimulation interferes with abnormal brain activity that occurs in PD. As a result there is significant improvement of the motor symptoms of PD (bradykinesia, rigidity, and tremor) as well as motor fluctuations and dyskinesias. This device can be turned off and on by a programming device or an external magnet.

The patient remains awake during most of the operative procedure so that he or she may respond to questions by the surgical team as the electrode is being advanced and stimulated. This is to be sure that the electrode is being correctly placed and that injury to other areas of the brain has not occurred. Patients may report unusual transient sensations including tingling, flashing lights, and changes in mood. Patients may also be able to report a decrease in symptoms.

Microelectrode and/or semimicroelectrode recording during the procedure allow precise physiological localization of a target region. Each time a new structure is encountered, a different physiological "signature" can be decoded.

Imaging plays an important role in localization of the target. MRI is used most often. CT is used when a patient cannot have an MRI, for example, if there is metal in the patient's body. A stereotactic surgical frame is attached to the patient's head to prevent any movement as the electrode is being carefully guided.

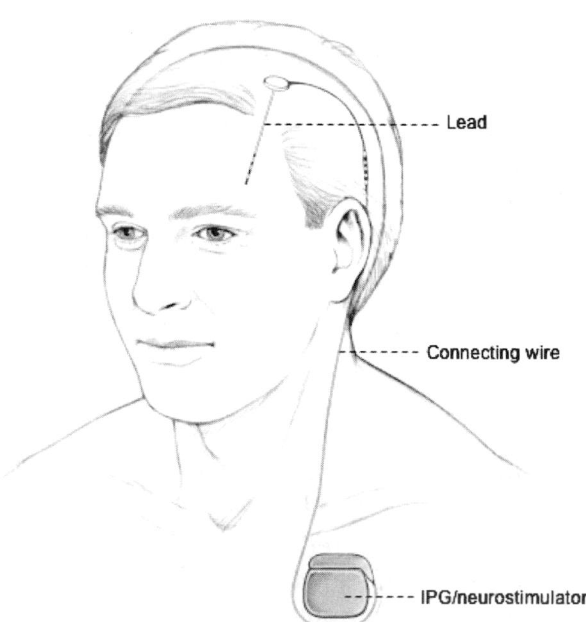

Figure 3.2 Showing a deep brain stimulator implanted with the battery
Note. Picture courtesy of Dr. Michael Okun, University of Florida

After the DBS electrode is implanted at its final location, it is secured to the skull with a specialized plastic burr-hole cover (or alternate securing mechanism) and the redundant electrode is buried under the scalp.

Under anesthesia, and commonly in a separate, staged procedure, a programmable pulse generator is implanted in a subcutaneous pocket under the clavicle.

An extension cable is then tunneled under the skin from the pulse generator to the scalp and connected to the implanted DBS electrode to complete the DBS system (see Figure 3.2).

Goals of DBS

- Reduce "off" time
- Reduce dyskinesias
- Smooth out motor fluctuations
- Possibly, reduce medication requirements

Patient Selection

Careful patient selection involves a rigorous screening process. It is preferable to have patients screened and worked up for PD surgery in an experienced and well-staffed multidisciplinary center because of the complex preoperative, intraoperative, and postoperative care required for these patients.

Screening includes:

- A comprehensive medical history and physical exam to confirm PD diagnosis, review symptoms, and assess therapeutic responses to date. A good medication and optimization trial should be implemented before scheduling a PD surgery.
- A discussion with the DBS neurologist to review what DBS is, what the goals of therapy are, and how this procedure relates to the patient and family support system.
- An evaluation of PD symptoms when off and on medications should be done. Patients should be evaluated with a Unified Parkinson's Disease Rating Scale (UPDRS) after abstaining from their medications the night prior to this evaluation. Section III of the UPDRS (the motor section) should be performed while the patient is off medications and then repeated while on medications. The on-off percentage difference should (in general) exceed 30% for the patient to be a reasonable candidate for surgery.

- A comprehensive neuropsychological workup to determine the patient's cognitive and mood state. Patients may also be referred for psychological assessment to assess coping strategies, discuss expectations of surgery, and evaluate support systems.
- Evaluation by the neurosurgeon, who will determine appropriateness for surgical candidacy, review procedure, and discuss risks in detail. Implanted hardware and devices will be reviewed. The surgical schedule will then be determined.

The Florida Surgical Questionnaire for Parkinson Disease (FLASQ-PD), a simple triage instrument for the general health care professional/neurologist, has been recently published. This instrument is a survey that can be filled out (in a few minutes' time) to aid in assessing surgical candidacy, and to assist in picking appropriate candidates for multidisciplinary surgical evaluations. The FLASQ-PD addresses diagnosis, red flags (characteristics making surgery potentially dangerous), favorable and unfavorable characteristics, medication trial, and exceptional circumstances such as a tremor that will not respond to medications. The instrument allows for a simple score to be awarded that will assess appropriateness of pursuing a full multidisciplinary PD surgical workup.

Characteristics of a Good Surgical Candidate

- A patient who is disabled by PD symptoms despite optimized medical therapy or who cannot tolerate medication side effects
- A patient whose target PD symptoms are dopamine responsive (i.e., bradykinesia, rigidity)
- A patient with reasonable expectations for surgery who understands that this is not a cure
- In most circumstances, a patient who is under 75 years of age, with a strong support system

Not a Good Surgical Candidate

- Causes of parkinsonism other than idiopathic PD, including all atypical and secondary parkinsonism
- Moderate to severe problems with dementia, anxiety, delusions, or depression
- Existing comorbidities
- Inability to cooperate during surgical procedure
- Lack of appropriate support system to assist with follow-up care

Risk of DBS

- 2%–3% risk of stroke or hemorrhage
- 4%–8% risk of infection, lead problems, skin breakdown
- Short-term changes in mental status; studies are ongoing to determine the long-term cognitive effects of DBS

Postoperative Concerns and Emergencies

- A change in the color of the skin that lies over the impulse generator or the lead could signify infection and patients should go to the hospital immediately for evaluation and/or antibiotics. Infections treated quickly and aggressively may obviate the need for device removal.
- Prolonged fever or drainage from the skin close to the device can also signify infection.
- Persistent confusion, disorientation, or mental status change can indicate infection, or other neurological emergencies.
- A rebound of symptoms can signify lead fractures or battery failure.
- Electric shocklike sensations can signify lead shorts.
- Sudden excessive spending of money, pressured talking, gambling, or grandiose behavior can signify mania.
- Feelings of doom, dysphoria, crying, and loss of energy may signify depression and should be treated quickly and aggressively because of the potentially increased risk of suicide in DBS.
- Tenseness, anxiety, and anger outbursts can all be the result of DBS.
- Persistent postoperative headaches can be a sign of hydrocephalus.
- Peri- and postoperative seizures can be a sign of hemorrhage, air, or subdural hematomas and should be followed up with immediate imaging studies.
- Device malfunction may occur at any time; sometimes the issue is as simple as an inadvertent turning off of the device by an external magnetic field. More concerning situations may include a fracture in the electrical connecting wires. Battery replacement is needed, on average, 3–5 years after the initial surgery.
- Caution is needed to ensure that individuals who undergo DBS surgery understand the risks that may occur to their device and should avoid exposure to MRI scanners and diathermy (e.g., heating pads). A Medtronic 24-hour phone line is available for

urgent questions: 800-707-0933; as well as information online at Medtronic.com.

Patient Follow-Up

- Each DBS program will have its own standard operating procedure for DBS follow-up. This includes a schedule of turning on the stimulator and follow-up programming. Suggestions from one center are listed below.

DBS Programming: General Concepts

- After activation, the DBS programmer can telemetrically set the device to one of thousands of different stimulation combinations.
- The device may be programmed and reprogrammed as many times as is needed.
- The stimulation parameters therefore can be adjusted to the needs of an individual patient.
- There may, however, be tradeoffs in programming the stimulator, as the site of optimal motor improvement may cause adverse cognitive or mood side effects.
- It is therefore of paramount importance that DBS centers place the devices into an optimal target location. Specifically, DBS leads should be implanted into the sensorimotor territories of the target nuclei (e.g., sensorimotor STN, GPi, thalamus), and care should be taken not to place the lead too close to surrounding anatomy, which may result in current spread and side effects.
- Leads placed in the nuclei, but causing current spread into limbic and associative regions, may cause further adverse mood and cognitive effects.
- Teams implanting and programming DBS devices should monitor the short- and long-term motor, mood, cognitive, and behavioral consequences of DBS.

Programming visits are likely to occur many times during the first 6 months, and then follow-up visits may be needed as frequently as every 6 months. There will be multiple adjustments in the stimulator and in the medications. There may be a reduction of medication doses in many, but not all patients.

SECTION IV

Appendices

Appendix I
Supplemental Reading

Bunting, L. K., & Vernon, G. M. (2007). *Comprehensive nursing care for Parkinson's disease.* New York: Springer.

Calne, S. M., & Kumar, A. (2003). Nursing care of patients with late-stage Parkinson's disease. *Journal of Neuroscience Nursing, 35,* 242–251.

Carter, J. H., Stewart, B. J., Archbold, P. G., Inoue, I., Jaglin, J., Lannon, M., et al. (1998). Living with a person who has Parkinson's disease: The spouses' perspective by stage of disease. *Movement Disorders, 13,* 20–28.

Chou, K. L., Evatt, M., Hinson, V., & Kompoliti, K. (2007). Sialorrhea in Parkinson's disease: A review. *Movement Disorders, 22,* 2306–2313.

Ellis, T., Katz, D. I., White, D. K., DePiero, T. J., Hohler, A. D., & Saint-Hilaire, M. H. (2008). Effectiveness of an inpatient multidisciplinary rehabilitation program for patients with Parkinson's disease. *Physical Therapy, 88*(7), 1–8.

Emre, M., Aarsland, D., Albanese, A., Byrne, E. J., Deuschl, G., De Deyn, P. P., et al. (2004). Rivastigmine for dementia associated with Parkinson's disease. *New England Journal of Medicine, 351,* 2509–2518.

Evans, A. H., Katzenschlager, R., Paviour, D., O'Sullivan, J. D., Appel, S., Lawrence, A. D., et al. (2004). Punding in Parkinson's disease: Its relation to the dopamine dysregulation syndrome. *Movement Disorders, 19,* 397–405.

Fernandez, H. H., & Friedman, J. H. (1999). Punding on L-dopa. *Movement Disorders, 14,* 836–838.

Friedman, J. H. (2008). *Making the connection between brain and behavior: Coping with Parkinson's disease.* New York: Demos Health.

Friedman, J. H., & Fernandez, H. H. (2000). Non-motor problems in Parkinson's disease. *Neurology, 6*(1), 18–27.

Hanagasi, H. A., & Emre, M. (2005). Treatment of behavioural symptoms and dementia in Parkinson's disease. *Fundamental and Clinical Pharmacology, 19,* 133–146.

Holden, K. (2000). *Parkinson's disease: Guidelines for medical nutrition therapy.* Fort Collins, CO: Five Star Living.

Keus, S. H. J., Bloem, B., Hendricks, E. J., Bredero-Cohen, A. B., Munneke, M., & Practice Recommendations Development Group. (2007). Evidence-based analysis of physical therapy in Parkinson's disease with recommendations for practice and research. *Movement Disorders, 22*(4), 451–460.

Loew, J. E., & Pratt, C. (2007). *Good nutrition and Parkinson's disease.* New York: American Parkinson's Disease Association.

Lyons, K. S., Stewart, B. J., Archbold, P. G., Carter, J. H., & Perrin, N. A. (2004). Pessimism and optimism as early warning signs for health decline in Parkinson's disease caregivers. *Nursing Research, 53,* 354–362.

Marjama-Lyons, J. M., & Koller, W. C. (2001). Parkinson's disease: Update in diagnosis and symptom management. *Geriatrics, 56,* 24–35.

Meyer, M. M., Derr, P., & Imke, S. (2007). *The comfort of home for Parkinson's disease: A guide for caregivers.* Portland, OR: Care Trust Publications.

Miyasaki, J. M, Martin, W., Suchowersky, O., Weiner, W. J., & Lang, A. E. (2002). Practice parameter: Initiation of treatment for Parkinson's disease: An evidence-based review. Report of the Quality Standards Subcommittee of the American Academy of Neurology. *Neurology, 58,* 11–17.

Muller, T. (2002). Drug treatment of non-motor symptoms in Parkinson's disease. *Expert Opinion in Pharmacotherapy, 3,* 381–388.

Okun, M. S., Fernandez, H. H., Rodriguez, R. L., & Foote, K. D. (2007). Identifying candidates for deep brain stimulation in Parkinson's disease: The role of the primary care physician. *Geriatrics, 62*(5), 18–24.

Okun, M. S., Rodriguez, R. L., Foote, K. D., Sudhyadhom, A., Bova, F., Jacobson, C., et al. (2008). A case-based review of troubleshooting deep brain stimulator issues in movement and neuropsychiatric disorders. *Parkinsonism and Related Disorders, 14*(7), 532–538.

Rabinstein, A. A, & Shulman, L. M. (2000). Management of behavioral and psychiatric problems in Parkinson's disease. *Parkinsonism and Related Disorders, 7,* 41–50.

Ravina, B., Putt, M., Siderowf, A., Farrar, J. T., Gillespie, M., Crawley, A., et al. (2005). Donepezil for dementia in Parkinson's disease: A randomized, double-blind, placebo-controlled, crossover study. *Journal of Neurology, Neurosurgery and Psychiatry, 76*(7), 934–939.

Rodriguez, R. L., Fernandez, H. H., Haq, I., & Okun, M. S. (2007). Pearls in patient selection for deep brain stimulation. *The Neurologist, 5,* 253–260.

Shapiro, M. A., Chang, Y. L., Munson, S. K., Jacobson IV, C. E., Rodriguez, R. L., Skidmore, F. M., et al. (2007). The 4 "A"s associated with pathological Parkinson gamblers: Anxiety, anger, age and agonists. *Neuropsychiatric Disease and Treatment, 3*(2), 1–7.

Uc, E. Y., Struck, L. K., Rodnitzky, R. L., Zimmerman, B., Dobson, J., Evans, W. J. (2006). Predictors of weight loss in Parkinson's disease. *Movement Disorders, 21*(7), 930–936.

Voon, V., Hassan, K., Zurowski, M., de Souza, M., Thomsen, T., Fox, S., et al. (2006). Prevalence of repetitive and reward-seeking behaviors in Parkinson disease. *Neurology, 67,* 1254–1257.

Waters, C. H. (2002). Treatment of advanced stage patients with Parkinson's disease. *Parkinsonism and Related Disorders, 9,* 15–21.

Zahodne, L. B., & Fernandez, H. H. (2006). Course prognosis and management of psychosis in Parkinson's disease: Are current treatments really effective? *CNS Spectrums, 13*(3)(Suppl. 4), 26–34.

Zahodne, L. B., & Fernandez, H. H. (2008). Pathophysiology and treatment of psychosis in Parkinson's disease: A review. *Drugs and Aging, 25*(8), 665–682.

Appendix II
Rating/Assessment Scales

Unified Parkinson Disease Rating Scale (UPDRS)

Part I. Mentation, Behavior, Mood

1 *Intellectual Impairment*
- 0 - none
- 1 - mild (consistent forgetfulness with partial recollection of events with no other difficulties)
- 2 - moderate memory loss with disorientation and moderate difficulty handling complex problems
- 3 - severe memory loss with disorientation to time and often place, severe impairment with problems
- 4 - severe memory loss with orientation only to person, unable to make judgments or solve problems

2 *Thought Disorder*
- 0 - none
- 1 - vivid dreaming
- 2 - "benign" hallucination with insight retained
- 3 - occasional to frequent hallucination or delusions without insight, could interfere with daily activities
- 4 - persistent hallucination, delusions, or florid psychosis

3 *Depression*
- 0 - not present
- 1 - periods of sadness or guilt greater than normal, never sustained for more than a few days or a week
- 2 - sustained depression for >1 week
- 3 - vegetative symptoms (insomnia, anorexia, abulia, weight loss)
- 4 - vegetative symptoms with suicidality

4 *Motivation/Initiative*
0 - normal
1 - less of assertive, more passive
2 - loss of initiative or disinterest in elective activities
3 - loss of initiative or disinterest in day-to-day (routine) activities
4 - withdrawn, complete loss of motivation

Part II. Activities of Daily Living

5 *Speech*
0 - normal
1 - mildly affected, no difficulty being understood
2 - moderately affected, may be asked to repeat
3 - severely affected, frequently asked to repeat
4 - unintelligible most of time

6 *Salivation*
0 - normal
1 - slight but noticeable increase, may have nighttime drooling
2 - moderately excessive saliva, daytime minimal drooling
3 - marked drooling

7 *Swallowing*
0 - normal
1 - rare choking
2 - occasional choking
3 - requires soft food
4 - requires NG tube or G tube

8 *Handwriting*
0 - normal
1 - slightly small or slow
2 - all words small but legible
3 - severely affected, not all words legible
4 - majority illegible

9 *Cutting Food/Handing Utensils*
0 - normal
1 - somewhat slow and clumsy but no help needed
2 - can cut most foods, some help needed
3 - food must be cut, but can feed self
4 - needs to be fed

10 *Dressing*
0 - normal
1 - somewhat slow, no help needed
2 - occasional help with buttons or arms in sleeves
3 - considerable help required but can do something alone
4 - helpless

11 *Hygiene*
0 - normal
1 - somewhat slow but no help needed
2 - needs help with shower or bath or very slow in hygienic care
3 - requires assistance for washing, brushing teeth, going to bathroom
4 - helpless

12 *Turning in Bed/Adjusting Bedclothes*
0 - normal
1 - somewhat slow, no help needed
2 - can turn alone or adjust sheets but with great difficulty
3 - can initiate but not turn or adjust alone
4 - helpless

13 *Falling—Unrelated to Freezing*
0 - none
1 - rare falls
2 - occasional, less than once per day
3 - average of once per day
4 - more than once per day

14 *Freezing When Walking*
0 - normal
1 - rare, may have start hesitation
2 - occasional falls from freezing
3 - frequent freezing, occasional falls
4 - frequent falls from freezing

15 *Walking*
0 - normal
1 - mild difficulty, day drag legs or decrease arm swing
2 - moderate difficulty, requires no assist
3 - severe disturbance, requires assistance
4 - cannot walk at all even with assist

16 *Tremor*

0 - absent
1 - slight and infrequent, not bothersome to patient
2 - moderate, bothersome to patient
3 - severe, interferes with many activities
4 - marked, interferes with many activities

17 *Sensory Complaints Related to Parkinsonism*

0 - none
1 - occasionally has numbness, tingling, and mild aching
2 - frequent, but not distressing
3 - frequent painful sensation
4 - excruciating pain

Part III. Motor Examination

18 *Speech*

0 - normal
1 - slight loss of expression, diction, and/or volume
2 - monotone, slurred but understandable, moderately impaired
3 - marked impairment, difficult to understand
4 - unintelligible

19 *Facial Expression*

0 - Normal
1 - minimal hypomimia, could be normal "poker face"
2 - slight but definite abnormal diminution in expression
3 - moderate hypomimia, lips parted some of time
4 - masked or fixed faces with severe or complete loss of facial expression, lips parted 1/4 inch or more

20 *Tremor at Rest*

a Face
b Right Upper Extremity
c Left Upper Extremity
d Right Lower Extremity
e Left Lower Extremity

0 - absent
1 - slight and infrequently present

2 - mild in amplitude and persistent, or moderate in amplitude, but only intermittently present
3 - moderate in amplitude and present most of time
4 - marked in amplitude and present most of time

21 *Action or Postural Tremor*

a Right Upper Extremity
b Left Upper Extremity

0 - absent
1 - slight, present with action
2 - moderate in amplitude, present with action
3 - moderate in amplitude, present with action and posture holding
4 - marked in amplitude, interferes with feeding

22 *Rigidity*

a Neck
b Right Upper Extremity
c Left Upper Extremity
d Right Lower Extremity
e Left Lower Extremity

0 - absent
1 - slight or detectable only with activation
2 - mild/moderate
3 - marked, but full range of motion easily achieved
4 - severe, range of motion achieved with difficulty

23 *Finger taps*

a Right
b Left

0 - normal
1 - mild slowing, and/or reduction in amplitude
2 - moderately impaired. Definite and early fatiguing, may have occasional arrests in movement
3 - severely impaired. Frequent hesitation in initiating movement or arrests in ongoing movement
4 - can barely perform the task

24 *Hand Movements (open and close hands in rapid succession)*
- **a** Right
- **b** Left

0 - normal
1 - mild slowing, and/or reduction in amplitude
2 - moderately impaired. Definite and early fatiguing, may have occasional arrests in movement
3 - severely impaired. Frequent hesitation in initiating movement or arrests in ongoing movement
4 - can barely perform the task

25 *Rapid Alternating Movements (pronate and supinate hands)*
- **a** Right
- **b** Left

0 - normal
1 - mild slowing, and/or reduction in amplitude
2 - moderately impaired. Definite and early fatiguing, may have occasional arrests in movement
3 - severely impaired. Frequent hesitation in initiating movement or arrests in ongoing movement
4 - can barely perform the task

26 *Leg Agility (tap heel on ground, amplitude should be 3 inches)*
- **a** Right
- **b** Left

0 - normal
1 - mild slowing, and/or reduction in amplitude
2 - moderately impaired. Definite and early fatiguing, may have occasional arrests in movement
3 - severely impaired. Frequent hesitation in initiating movement or arrests in ongoing movement
4 - can barely perform the task

27 *Arising From Chair (patient arises with arms folded across chest)*
0 - normal
1 - slow, may need more than one attempt
2 - pushes self up from arms or seat
3 - tends to fall back, may need multiple tries but can arise without assistance
4 - unable to arise without help

28 *Posture*
0 - normal erect
1 - not quite erect, slightly stooped, could be normal for older person
2 - moderately stooped, definitely abnormal, may lean to one side
3 - severely stooped with kyphosis, can be moderately leaning to one side
4 - marked flexion with extreme abnormality of posture

29 *Gait*
0 - normal
1 - walks slowly, may shuffle with short steps, no festination or propulsion
2 - walks with difficulty, but requires little or no assistance, may have some festination, short steps or propulsion
3 - severe disturbance of gait requiring assistance
4 - cannot walk at all, even with assistance

30 *Postural Stability (retropulsion test)*
0 - normal
1 - retropulsion, but recovers unaided
2 - absence of postural response, would fall if not caught by examiner
3 - very unstable, tends to lose balance spontaneously
4 - unable to stand without assistance

31 *Body Bradykinesia/Hypokinesia*
0 - none
1 - minimal slowness, giving movement a deliberate character, could be normal for some persons, possibly reduced amplitude
2 - mild degree of slowness and poverty of movement, definitely abnormal, alternatively some reduced amplitude
3 - moderate slowness, poverty, or small amplitude of movement
4 - marked slowness, poverty, or amplitude of movement

Part IV. Complications of Therapy

A. Dyskinesias

32 *Duration (What proportion of the waking day are dyskinesias present?)*
0 - none
1 - 1%–25% of day

2 - 26%–50% of day
3 - 51%–75% of day
4 - 76%–100% of day

33 *Disability (How disabling are the dyskinesias?)*
0 - not disabling
1 - mildly disabling
2 - moderately disabling
3 - severly disabling
4 - completely disabling

34 *Painful dyskinesias (How painful are the dyskinesias?)*
0 - not painful
1 - slightly
2 - moderately
3 - severely
4 - markedly

35 *Presence of early morning dystonia (historical information)*
0 - no
1 - yes

B. Clinical Fluctuations

36 *Are any "off" periods predictable as to timing after a dose of medication?*
0 - no
1 - yes

37 *Are any "off" periods unpredictable as to timing after a dose of medication?*
0 - no
1 - yes

38 *Do any "off" periods come on suddenly (e.g., within a few seconds)?*
0 - no
1 - yes

39 *What proportion of the waking day is the subject "off" on average?*
0 - none
1 - 1%–25% of day
2 - 26%–50% of day
3 - 51%–75% of day
4 - 76%–100% of day

C. Other Complications

40 *Does the subject have anorexia, nausea, or vomiting?*
0 - no
1 - yes

41 *Does the subject have any sleep disturbances (e.g., insomnia or hypersomnolence)?*
0 - no
1 - yes

42 *Does the subject have symptomatic orthostasis?*
0 - no
1 - yes

Modified Hoehn and Yahr Scale

Stage 0	No signs of PD
Stage 1	Unilateral involvement only
Stage 1.5	Unilateral involvement and axial involvement
Stage 2	Bilateral involvement without impairment of balance
Stage 2.5	Bilateral involvement with recovery on retropulsion test
Stage 3	Mild to moderate bilateral involvement with some postural instability, but physically independent
Stage 4	Severe disability but still able to walk or stand unassisted
Stage 5	Wheelchair bound or bedridden unless aided

Schwab and England Activities of Daily Living Scale

100% = Completely independent. Able to do all chores without slowness, difficulty, or impairment. Essentially normal. Unaware of any difficulty.

90% = Completely independent. Able to do all chores with some degree of slowness, difficulty, and impairment. Might take twice as long. Beginning to be aware of difficulty.
80% = Completely independent in most chores. Takes twice as long. Conscious of difficulty and slowness.
70% = Not completely independent. More difficult with some chores. Three to four times as long in some. Must spend a large part of the day with chores.
60% = Some dependency. Can do most chores, but exceedingly slowly and with much effort. Errors; some chores impossible.
50% = More dependent. Help with half the chores, slower, and so forth. Difficulty with everything.
40% = Very dependent. Can assist with all chores, but few alone.
30% = With effort, now and then does a few chores alone or begins alone. Much help is needed.
20% = Nothing alone. Can be slight help with some chores. Severe invalid.
10% = Totally dependent, helpless. Complete invalid.
0% = Vegetative functions such as swallowing, bladder, and bowel functions are not functioning. Bedridden.

Florida Parkinson's Disease Surgery Questionnaire (FLASQ-PD)

A. Diagnosis of Idiopathic Parkinson's Disease

Diagnosis 1: Is bradykinesia present? Yes / No (Please circle response)

Diagnosis 2: *(check if present):*
___ Rigidity (Stiffness in arms, leg, or neck)
___ 4–6 Hertz resting tremor
___ Postural instability not caused by primary visual, vestibular, cerebellar, proprioceptive dysfunction

Does your patient have at least two of the above? Yes / No (Please circle response)

Diagnosis 3: *(check if present):*
___ Unilateral onset
___ Rest tremor present
___ Progressive disorder
___ Persistent asymmetry affecting side of onset most

___ Excellent response (70%–100%) to levodopa
___ Severe levodopa-induced dyskinesia
___ Levodopa response for 5 years or more
___ Clinical course of 5 years or more

Does your patient have at least three of the above? Yes / No (Please circle response)

("Yes" answers to all three questions above suggest the diagnosis of idiopathic PD)

B. Findings Suggestive of Parkinsonism Caused by a Process Other Than Idiopathic PD

Primitive Reflexes
- 1 - RED FLAG–presence of a grasp, snout, root, suck, or Myerson's sign
- N/A–not done/unknown

Presence of supranuclear gaze palsy
- 1 - RED FLAG–supranuclear gaze palsy present
- N/A–not done/unknown

Presence of ideomotor apraxia
- 1 - RED FLAG–ideomotor apraxia present
- N/A–not done/unknown

Presence of autonomic dysfunction
- 1 - RED FLAG–presence of new severe orthostatic hypotension not caused by medications, erectile dysfunction, or other autonomic disturbance within the first year or two of disease onset
- N/A–not done/unknown

Presence of a wide-based gait
- 1 - RED FLAG–wide-based gait present
- N/A–not done/unknown

Presence of more than mild dementia
- 1 - RED FLAG–frequently disoriented or severe cognitive difficulties or severe memory problems, or anomia
- N/A–not done, not known

Presence of severe psychosis
- 1 - RED FLAG–presence of severe psychosis, refractory to medications
- N/A–not done, not known

History of unresponsiveness to levodopa

1 - RED FLAG–Parkinsonism is clearly not responsive to levodopa, or patient is dopamine naïve, or patient has not had a trial of levodopa
N/A–not done, not known

(Any of the "FLAGs" above may be contraindications to surgery)

C. Patient Characteristics *(Circle the one best answer that characterizes your Parkinson's Disease Surgical Candidate):*

1 Age:
0 - >80
1 - 71–80
2 - 61–70
3 - <61

2 Duration of Parkinson's symptoms:
0 - <3 years
1 - 4–5 years
2 - >5 years

3 On-Off fluctuations (medications wear off, fluctuate with dyskinesia and akinesia)?
0 - no
1 - yes

4 Dyskinesias
0 - none
1 - <50% of the time
2 - >50% of the time

5 Dystonia
0 - none
1 - <50% of the time
2 - >50% of the time

General Patient Characteristics Subscore ____

D. Favorable/Unfavorable Characteristics

6 Gait Freezing
0 - not responsive to levodopa during the best "on"
1 - responsive to levodopa during the best "on"
NA–not applicable

7 Postural Instability
0 - not responsive to levodopa during the best "on"
1 - responsive to levodopa during the best "on"
NA–not applicable

8 Warfarin or other blood thinners
   0 - on warfarin or another blood thinner besides antiplatelet therapy
   1 - not on warfarin or another blood thinner besides antiplatelet therapy

9 Cognitive function:
   0 - memory difficulties or frontal deficits
   1 - no signs or symptoms of cognitive dysfunction

10 Swallowing function
   0 - frequent choking or aspiration
   1 - occasional choking
   2 - rare choking
   3 - no swallowing difficulties

11 Continence
   0 - incontinent of bowel and bladder
   1 - incontinent of bladder only
   2 - no incontinence

12 Depression
   0 - severe depression with vegetative symptoms
   1 - treated, moderate depression
   2 - mild depressive symptoms
   3 - no depression

13 Psychosis:
   0 - frequent hallucinations
   1 - occasional hallucinations (probably medication-related)
   2 - no hallucinations

Favorable/Unfavorable Characteristics Subscore ____

E. Medication Trials *(circle the best answer)*

14 Historical response to levodopa:
   0 - uncertain historical response to levodopa, or no trial of levodopa
   1 - history of modest improvement with levodopa
   2 - history of marked improvement with levodopa

15 Trial of Sinemet (carbidopa/levodopa or Madopar or equivalent):
   0 - No trial or less than three times a day
   1 - Sinemet three times a day
   2 - Sinemet four times a day
   3 - Sinemet greater than four times a day

16 Trial of Dopamine Agonist:
0 - No trial or less than three times a day
1 - Dopamine Agonist three times a day
2 - Dopamine Agonist four times a day
3 - Dopamine Agonist greater than four times a day

17 Trial of Sinemet Extender
0 - No trial
1 - Trial of either tolcapone or entacapone

18 Trial of a combination of Sinemet or equivalent with a dopamine agonist
0 - No trial
1 - Trial of Sinemet or equivalent with a dopamine agonist

Medication Trial Subscore: _____

FLASQ-PD Scoring:

A. Met Diagnostic Criteria of Idiopathic PD: Yes / No
B. Contraindications (FLAGS) Subscore: ____ (8 possible; any flags = likely not a good candidate)
C. General Characteristics Subscore ____ (10 possible)
D. Favorable/Unfavorable Characteristics Subscore: ____ (14 possible)
E. Medication Trial Subscore ____ (10 possible)

Total Scale Score (C+D+E): ____ (34 possible)

Presence of Refractory Tremor: Yes / No (Presence of moderate to severe tremor that is refractory to high doses and combinations of levodopa, dopamine agonists, and anticholinergics may be an indication for surgery in some candidates, independent of their score on the remainder of the questionnaire)

F. Abnormal Involuntary Movement Scale

Instructions: Complete the examination procedure before making ratings. When rating movements, rate the highest severity observed and rate movements that occur upon activation one less than those observed spontaneously

Facial and Oral Movements

1 Muscles of facial expression (e.g., movement of forehead, eyebrows, periorbital area, cheeks; include frowning, blinking, smiling, grimacing)
  1 None, normal
  2 Minimal
  3 Mild
  4 Moderate
  5 Severe

☐

2 Lips and perioral area (e.g., puckering, pouting, smacking)
  1 None, normal
  2 Minimal
  3 Mild
  4 Moderate
  5 Severe

☐

3 Jaws (e.g., biting, clenching, chewing, mouth opening, lateral movement)
  1 None, normal
  2 Minimal
  3 Mild
  4 Moderate
  5 Severe

☐

4 Tongue (rate only increase in movement both in and out of mouth, *not* inability to sustain movement)
  1 None, normal
  2 Minimal
  3 Mild
  4 Moderate
  5 Severe

☐

Extremity Movements

5 Upper (arms, wrists, hands, fingers). Include choreic movements (i.e., rapid, objectively purposeless, irregular, spontaneous), athetoid movements (i.e., slow, irregular, complex, serpentine). Do NOT include tremor (i.e., repetitive, regular, rhythmic).

1 None, normal
2 Minimal
3 Mild
4 Moderate
5 Severe

6 Lower (legs, knees, ankles, toes, e.g., lateral knee movement, foot tapping, heel dropping, foot squirming, inversion and eversion of foot)
   1 None, normal
   2 Minimal
   3 Mild
   4 Moderate
   5 Severe

Trunk Movements

7 Neck, shoulders, hips (e.g., rocking, twisting, squirming, pelvic gyrations)
   1 None, normal
   2 Minimal
   3 Mild
   4 Moderate
   5 Severe

Global Judgments

8 Severity of abnormal movements
   1 None, normal
   2 Minimal
   3 Mild
   4 Moderate
   5 Severe

9 Incapacitation due to abnormal movements
   1 None, normal
   2 Minimal
   3 Mild
   4 Moderate
   5 Severe

10 Patient's awareness of abnormal movements (rate only patient's report)

1 No awareness
2 Aware, no distress
3 Aware, mild distress
4 Aware, moderate distress
5 Aware, severe distress

☐

Dental Status

11 Current problems with teeth and/or dentures

1 No
2 Yes

☐

12 Does patient usually wear dentures?

1 No
2 Yes

☐

G. Epworth Sleepiness Scale

Use the following scale to choose the most appropriate number for each situation:
0 = would *never* doze or sleep.
1 = *slight* chance of dozing or sleeping
2 = *moderate* chance of dozing or sleeping
3 = *high* chance of dozing or sleeping

Situation	***Chance of Dozing or Sleeping***
Sitting and reading	____
Watching TV	____
Sitting inactive in a public place	____
Being a passenger in a motor vehicle for an hour or more	____
Lying down in the afternoon	____
Sitting and talking to someone	____
Sitting quietly after lunch (no alcohol)	____
Stopped for a few minutes in traffic while driving	____
Total score (add up the scores)	____

H. Parkinson's Disease Sleep Scale

Parkinson's Disease Sleep Scale			
1	The overall quality of your night's sleep is	AWFUL	EXCELLENT
2	Do you have difficulty falling asleep at night?	ALWAYS	NEVER
3	Do you have difficulty staying asleep?	ALWAYS	NEVER
4	Do you have restlessness of legs or arms at night or in the evening, causing disruption of sleep?	ALWAYS	NEVER
5	Do you fidget in bed?	ALWAYS	NEVER
6	Do you suffer from distressing dreams at night?	ALWAYS	NEVER
7	Do you suffer from distressing hallucinations at night (seeing or hearing things that you are told do not exist)?	ALWAYS	NEVER
8	Do you get up at night to pass urine?	ALWAYS	NEVER
9	Do you have incontinence of urine because you are unable to move due to 'off' symptoms?	ALWAYS	NEVER
10	Do you experience numbness or tingling of your arms or legs which wake you from sleep at night?	ALWAYS	NEVER
11	Do you have painful muscle cramps in your arms or legs while sleeping at night?	ALWAYS	NEVER
12	Do you wake early in the morning with painful posturing of arms or legs?	ALWAYS	NEVER
13	On waking, do you experience tremor?	ALWAYS	NEVER
14	Do you feel tired and sleepy after waking in the morning?	ALWAYS	NEVER
15	Have you unexpectedly fallen asleep during the day?	FREQUENTLY	NEVER

I. Parkinson's Disease Questionnaire (PDQ-39)

Instructions: Please read the following statements and check one box for each question. **On account of your movement disorder, how often during the *last month* have you...**

	Never	Occasionally	Sometimes	Often	Always or cannot do
1. Had difficulty doing the leisure activities you like?	☐	☐	☐	☐	☐
2. Had difficulty looking after your home, e.g., housework, cooking?	☐	☐	☐	☐	☐
3. Had difficulty carrying shopping bags?	☐	☐	☐	☐	☐
4. Had problems walking half a mile?	☐	☐	☐	☐	☐
5. Had problems walking 100 yards?	☐	☐	☐	☐	☐
6. Had problems getting around the house as easily as you would like?	☐	☐	☐	☐	☐
7. Had difficulty getting around in public places?	☐	☐	☐	☐	☐
8. Needed someone to accompany you when you went out?	☐	☐	☐	☐	☐
9. Felt frightened or worried about falling over in public?	☐	☐	☐	☐	☐
10. Been confined to the house more than you would like?	☐	☐	☐	☐	☐
11. Had difficulty washing yourself?	☐	☐	☐	☐	☐
12. Avoided situations that involve eating or drinking in public?	☐	☐	☐	☐	☐
13. Felt embarrassed in public due to your medical condition?	☐	☐	☐	☐	☐

Parkinson's Disease Questionnaire (PDQ-39) (Continued)

14. Felt worried about people's reactions to you?	☐	☐	☐	☐	☐
15. Had problems with your close personal relationships?	☐	☐	☐	☐	☐
16. Not had support in the ways you need from your spouse or partner?	☐	☐	☐	☐	☐
17. Not had support in the ways you need from your family or close friends?	☐	☐	☐	☐	☐
18. Unexpectedly fallen asleep during the day?	☐	☐	☐	☐	☐
19. Had problems with your concentration, e.g., when reading or watching TV?	☐	☐	☐	☐	☐
20. Felt your memory was bad?	☐	☐	☐	☐	☐
21. Had distressing dreams or hallucinations?	☐	☐	☐	☐	☐
22. Had difficulty with your speech?	☐	☐	☐	☐	☐
23. Felt unable to communicate with people property?	☐	☐	☐	☐	☐
24. Felt ignored by people?	☐	☐	☐	☐	☐
25. Had painful muscle spasms?	☐	☐	☐	☐	☐
26. Had aches and pains in your joints or body?	☐	☐	☐	☐	☐
27. Felt unpleasantly hot or cold?	☐	☐	☐	☐	☐

J. Brief Psychiatric Rating Scale

Instructions: Please enter the score for the term that best describes the patient's condition.				
1 = not present 2 = very mild	3 = mild 4 = moderate	5 = moderately severe 6 = severe	7 = extremely severe N = not assessed	
				Rating:
1. SOMATIC CONCERN–preoccupation with physical health, fear of physical illness, hypochondriasis				
2. ANXIETY–worry, fear, overconcern for present or future				
3. EMOTIONAL WITHDRAWAL–no spontaneous interaction, isolation, deficiency in relating to others				
4. CONCEPTUAL DISORGANIZATION–confused, disconnected, disorganized, disrupted				
5. GUILT FEELINGS–self-blame shame, remorse for past				
6. TENSION–physical and motor manifestations of nervousness, overactivation, tension				
7. MANNERISMS & POSTURING–peculiar, bizarre, unnatural motor behavior				
8. GRANDIOSITY–exaggerated self-opinion, arrogance, conviction of unusual power or abilities				
9. DEPRESSIVE MOOD–sorrow, sadness, despondency, pessimism				
10. HOSTILITY–animosity, contempt, belligerence, disdain for others				
11. SUSPICIOUSNESS–mistrust, belief others harbor malicious or discriminatory intent				
12. HALLUCINATIONS–perceptions without normal external stimulus correspondence				
13. MOTOR RETARDATION–slowed weakened movements or speech, reduced body tone				
14. UNCOOPERATIVENESS–resistance, guardedness, rejection of authority				
15. UNUSUAL THOUGHT CONTENT–unusual, odd, strange, bizarre thought content				
16. BLUNTED AFFECT–reduced emotional tone, reduction in normal intensity of feelings, flatness				
17. EXCITEMENT–heightened emotional tone, agitation, increased reactivity				
18. DISORIENTATION–confusion or lack of proper association for person, place, or time				

K. Neuropsychiatric Inventory Questionnaire

Name of patient: ______________________________ Date: ____________

Informant: Spouse: ___________ Child: _________ Other: _____________

Please answer the following questions based on *changes* that have occurred since the patient first began to experience memory problems.

Circle "yes" only if the symptom has been present in the *past month*. Otherwise, circle "no."

For each item marked "yes":

Rate the *severity* of the symptom (how it affects the patient):

1 = Mild (noticeable, but not a significant change)
2 = Moderate (significant, but not a dramatic change)
3 = Severe (very marked or prominent; a dramatic change)

Rate the distress you experience because of that symptom (how it affects you):

0 = Not distressing at all
1 = Minimal (slightly distressing, not a problem to cope with)
2 = Mild (not very distressing, generally easy to cope with)
3 = Moderate (fairly distressing, not always easy to cope with)
4 = Severe (very distressing, difficult to cope with)
5 = Extreme or very severe (extremely distressing, unable to cope with)

Please answer each question honestly and carefully. Ask for assistance if you are not sure how to answer any question.

Delusions		Does the patient believe that others are stealing from him or her, or planning to harm him or her in some way?	
Yes	No	Severity: 1 2 3	Distress: 0 1 2 3 4 5
Hallucinations		Does the patient act as if he or she hears voices? Does he or she talk to people who are not there?	
Yes	No	Severity: 1 2 3	Distress: 0 1 2 3 4 5
Agitation or aggression		Is the patient stubborn and resistive to help from others?	
Yes	No	Severity: 1 2 3	Distress: 0 1 2 3 4 5

Depression or dysphoria Yes No	Does the patient act as if he or she is sad or in low spirits? Does he or she cry? Severity: 1 2 3 Distress: 0 1 2 3 4 5
Anxiety Yes No	Does the patient become upset when separated from you? Does he or she have any other signs of nervousness, such as shortness of breath, sighing, being unable to relax, or feeling excessively tense? Severity: 1 2 3 Distress: 0 1 2 3 4 5
Elation or euphoria Yes No	Does the patient appear to feel too good or act excessively happy? Severity: 1 2 3 Distress: 0 1 2 3 4 5
Apathy or indifference Yes No	Does the patient seem less interested in his or her usual activities and in the activities and plans of others? Severity: 1 2 3 Distress: 0 1 2 3 4 5
Disinhibition Yes No	Does the patient seem to act impulsively? For example, does the patient talk to strangers as if he or she knows them, or does the patient say things that may hurt people's feelings? Severity: 1 2 3 Distress: 0 1 2 3 4 5
Irritability or lability Yes No	Is the patient impatient and cranky? Does he or she have difficulty coping with delays or waiting for planned activities? Severity: 1 2 3 Distress: 0 1 2 3 4 5
Motor disturbance Yes No	Does the patient engage in repetitive activities, such as pacing around the house, handling buttons, wrapping string, or doing other things repeatedly? Severity: 1 2 3 Distress: 0 1 2 3 4 5
Nighttime behaviors Yes No	Does the patient awaken you during the night, rise too early in the morning, or take excessive naps during the day? Severity: 1 2 3 Distress: 0 1 2 3 4 5
Appetite and eating Yes No	Has the patient lost or gained weight, or had a change in the food he or she likes? Severity: 1 2 3 Distress: 0 1 2 3 4 5

L. Geriatric Depression Scale (Original 30-Item Version)

Choose the best answer for how you have felt over the past week:

1. Are you basically satisfied with your life? YES / NO
2. Have you dropped many of your activities and interests? YES / NO
3. Do you feel that your life is empty? YES / NO
4. Do you often get bored? YES / NO
5. Are you hopeful about the future? YES / NO
6. Are you bothered by thoughts you can't get out of your head? YES / NO
7. Are you in good spirits most of the time? YES / NO
8. Are you afraid that something bad is going to happen to you? YES / NO
9. Do you feel happy most of the time? YES / NO
10. Do you often feel helpless? YES / NO
11. Do you often get restless and fidgety? YES / NO
12. Do you prefer to stay at home, rather than going out and doing new things? YES / NO
13. Do you frequently worry about the future? YES / NO
14. Do you feel you have more problems with memory than most? YES / NO
15. Do you think it is wonderful to be alive now? YES / NO
16. Do you often feel downhearted and blue? YES / NO
17. Do you feel pretty worthless the way you are now? YES / NO
18. Do you worry a lot about the past? YES / NO
19. Do you find life very exciting? YES / NO
20. Is it hard for you to get started on new projects? YES / NO
21. Do you feel full of energy? YES / NO
22. Do you feel that your situation is hopeless? YES / NO
23. Do you think that most people are better off than you are? YES / NO
24. Do you frequently get upset over little things? YES / NO
25. Do you frequently feel like crying? YES / NO
26. Do you have trouble concentrating? YES / NO
27. Do you enjoy getting up in the morning? YES / NO
28. Do you prefer to avoid social gatherings? YES / NO
29. Is it easy for you to make decisions? YES / NO
30. Is your mind as clear as it used to be? YES / NO

Scoring instructions: One point for each of these answers. Cutoff: normal, 0–9; mild depressives, 10–19; severe depressives, 20–30.

1. no	6. yes	11. yes	16. yes	21. no	26. yes
2. yes	7. no	12. yes	17. yes	22. yes	27. no
3. yes	8. yes	13. yes	18. yes	23. yes	28. yes
4. yes	9. no	14. yes	19. no	24. yes	29. no
5. no	10. yes	15. no	20. yes	25. yes	30. no

M. Geriatric Depression Scale (Short Version)

Choose the best answer for how you have felt over the past week:

1 Are you basically satisfied with your life? YES / **NO**
2 Have you dropped many of your activities and interests? **YES** / NO
3 Do you feel that your life is empty? **YES** / NO
4 Do you often get bored? **YES** / NO
5 Are you in good spirits most of the time? YES / **NO**
6 Are you afraid that something bad is going to happen to you? **YES** / NO
7 Do you feel happy most of the time? YES / **NO**
8 Do you often feel helpless? **YES** / NO
9 Do you prefer to stay at home, rather than going out and doing new things? **YES** / NO
10 Do you feel you have more problems with memory than most? **YES** / NO
11 Do you think it is wonderful to be alive now? YES / **NO**
12 Do you feel pretty worthless the way you are now? **YES** / NO
13 Do you feel full of energy? YES / **NO**
14 Do you feel that your situation is hopeless? **YES** / NO
15 Do you think that most people are better off than you are? **YES** / NO

Answers in **bold** indicate depression. Although differing sensitivities and specificities have been obtained across studies, for clinical purposes a score >5 points is suggestive of depression and should warrant a follow-up interview. Scores >10 are almost always depression.

N. Hamilton Depression Scale (HAM-D)

1. Depressed Mood (sadness, hopelessness, helplessness, worthlessness)
0 - Absent.
1 - These feeling states indicated only on questioning.
2 - These feeling states spontaneously reported verbally.
3 - Communicates feeling states nonverbally – i.e., through facial expression, posture, voice, and tendency to weep.
4 - Patient reports virtually only these feeling states in spontaneous verbal and nonverbal communication.

Score: 0 1 2 3 4

2. Feelings of Guilt
0 - Absent.
1 - Feels life is not worth living.
2 - Ideas of guilt or rumination over past errors or sinful deeds.
3 - Present illness is a punishment. Delusions of guilt.
4 - Hears accusatory or denouncing voices and/or experiences threatening visual hallucinations.

Score: 0 1 2 3 4

3. Suicide
0 - Absent.
1 - Self-reproach, feels she/he has let people down.
2 - Wishes she/he were dead or any thought of possible death to self.
3 - Suicide ideas or gesture.
4 - Attempts at suicide.

Score: 0 1 2 3 4

4. Insomnia – Early
0 - No difficulty falling asleep.
1 - Complains of occasional difficulty falling asleep – i.e., more than ½ hour.
2 - Complains of occasional nightly difficulty falling asleep.

Score: 0 1 2

5. Insomnia – Middle
0 - No difficulty.
1 - Patient complains of being restless and disturbed during the night.
2 - Waking during the night – gets out of bed.

Score: 0 1 2

6. Insomnia – Late
0 - Sleeps until awakened.
1 - Wakes in early hours of the morning but goes back to sleep.
2 - Unable to fall asleep again if gets out of bed.

Score: 0 1 2

7. Work and Activities
0 - No difficulty.
1 - Thoughts and feelings of incapacity, fatigue, or weakness related to activities, work, or hobbies.
2 - Loss of interest in activities, hobbies, or work – either directly reported by the patient or indirectly in listlessness, indecision, and vacillation (feels she/he has to push self to work or participate in activities).

Score: 0 1 2

8. Retardation (slowness of thought and speech: impaired ability to concentrate: decreased motor activity)
0 - Normal speech and thought.
1 - Slight retardation at interview.
2 - Obvious retardation at interview.
3 - Interview difficult.
4 - Complete stupor.

Score: 0 1 2 3 4

9. Agitation
0 - None.
1 - "Playing with" hands, hair, etc.
2 - Hand-wringing, nail-biting, hair pulling, biting of lips.

Score: 0 1 2

10. Anxiety – Psychic
0 - No difficulty.
1 - Subjective tension and irritability.
2 - Worrying about minor matters.
3 - Apprehensive attitude apparent in face or speech.
4 - Fears expressed without questioning.

Score: 0 1 2 3 4

11. Anxiety – Somatic Psychological concomitants of anxiety, such as:
Gastrointestinal – dry mouth, wind, indigestion, diarrhea, cramps, belching
Cardiovascular – palpitations, headaches
Respiratory – hyperventilation, sighing
Urinary frequency
Sweating
Rate severity of any or all at:
0 – Absent 1 – Mild 2 – Moderate 3 –Severe 4 – Incapacitating

Score: 0 1 2 3 4

12. Somatic Symptoms – Gastrointestinal
0 - None.
1 - Loss of appetite but eating without encouragement. Heavy feeling in abdomen.
2 - Difficulty eating without urging. Requests or requires laxative or medication for bowels or medication for G.I. symptoms.

Score: 0 1 2

13. Somatic Symptoms – General
0 - None.
1 - Heaviness in limbs, back, or head. Backaches, headaches, muscle aches. Loss of energy and fatigability.
2 - Any clear-cut symptom.

Score: 0 1 2

14. Genital Symptoms (such as loss of libido, menstrual disturbances, etc.)
0 - Absent.
1 - Mild.
2 - Severe.

Score: 0 1 2

15. Hypochondriasis
0 - Not present.
1 - Self-absorption (bodily).
2 - Preoccupation with health.
3 - Frequent complaints, requests for help, etc.
4 - Hypochondriacal delusions.

Score: 0 1 2 3 4

16. Loss of Weight
A. Rating by history:
0 - No weight loss.
1 - Probably weight loss associated with present illness.
2 - Definite (according to patient) weight loss.
B. Rating by actual weight change.
0 - Less than 1 lb. loss in week.
1 - One lb. or greater loss in week.
2 - Two lb. or greater loss in week.

Score A: 0 1 2 Score B: 0 1 2

17. Insight
0 - Acknowledges being depressed and ill.
1 - Acknowledges illness but attributes cause to bad food, climate, overwork, virus, need for rest, etc.
2 - Denies being ill at all.

Score: 0 1 2

References

Chaudhuri, K. R., Pal, S., DiMarco, A., Whately-Smith, C., Bridgman, K., Mathew, R., et al. (2002). The Parkinson's disease sleep scale: A new instrument for assessing sleep and nocturnal disability in Parkinson's disease. *Journal of Neurology, Neurosurgery, and Psychiatry, 73,* 629–635.

Cummings, J. L., Mega, M., Gray, K., Rosenberg-Thompson, S., Carusi, D. A., & Gornbein, J. (1994). The Neuropsychiatric Inventory: Comprehensive assessment of psychopathology in dementia. *Neurology, 44,* 2308–2314.

Fahn, S., & Elton, R. L. (1987). Members of the UPDRS Development Committee: Unified Parkinson's Disease Rating Scale. In S. Fahn, C. D. Marsden, D. B. Calne, & A. Lieberman (Eds.), *Recent developments in Parkinson's disease* (Vol. 2, pp. 153–163). Florham Park, NJ: Macmillan Health Care Information.

Hamilton, M. (1967). Development of a rating scale for primary depressive illness. *The British Journal of Social and Clinical Psychology, 6,* 278–296.

Hoehn, M. M., & Yahr, M. D. (1967). Parkinsonism: Onset, progression and mortality. *Neurology, 17,* 427–442.

Johns, M. W. (1991). A new method for measuring daytime sleepiness: The Epworth Sleepiness Scale. *Sleep, 14,* 540–545.

Okun, M. S., Fernandez, H. H., Pedraza, O., Misra, M., Lyons, K. E., Pahwa, R., et al. (2004). Development and initial validation of a screening tool for Parkinson Disease surgical candidates. *Neurology, 63,* 161 163.

Overall, J. E., & Gorham, D. R. (1962). The Brief Psychiatric Rating Scale. *Psychological Report, 10,* 799–812.

Peto, V., Jenkinson, C., Fitzpatrick, R., & Greenhall, R. (1995). The development of a short measure of functioning and well-being for individuals with Parkinson's disease. *Quality of Life Research, 4,* 241–248.

Psychopharmacology Research Branch, NIMH. (1976). Abnormal Involuntary Movement Scale (AIMS). In W. Guy (Ed.), *ECDEU assessment manual for Psychopharmacology* (rev. ed., pp. 534–537). DHEW Pub No (ADM) 76-338. Rockville, MD: National Institute of Mental Health.

Schwab, R. S., & England, A. C., Jr. (1969). Projection technique for evaluating surgery in Parkinson's disease. In F. J. Gilingham & I. M. L. Donaldson (Eds.), *Third symposium on Parkinson's disease* (pp. 152–157). Edinburgh, Scotland: E & S Livingstone.

Yesavage, J., Brink, T., Rose, T., Lum, O., Huang, V., Adey, M., et al. (1983). Development and validation of a geriatric depression screening scale: A preliminary report. *Journal of Psychiatric Research, 17,* 37–49.

Appendix III
Medication Tools

Medication Management of Individuals With Parkinson's Disease

Parkinson's disease is a movement disorder.
The primary symptoms of PD include:
Muscle Rigidity
Slowness of Movement (*Bradykinesia*)
Tremor (usually at rest)
Impaired Balance

Each person with PD has a unique set of symptoms and symptom severity that may change over time.
The path, or course, an individual follows over his/her lifetime with the disease is influenced by many factors including medication management.

The health care professional must begin the assessment process by working with the patient to identify each symptom that is present, how severe or bothersome each symptom is to the patient, and what is the daily pattern of each symptom. . . .

For example:
When does your (*symptom*) start?
When is your (*symptom*) at its worst?
How long does your (*symptom*) last?
How bad is your (*symptom*)?
Does your (*symptom*) happen every day?

Help the patient develop useful tools such as calendars, diaries, computer logs, etc.

IDENTIFY THE SYMPTOMS → ESTABLISH THE DAILY PATTERN OF SYMPTOMS

The primary objective of medication management is to maximize daily control over the symptoms of PD while preventing or limiting the occurrence of side effects.

Each medication is selected for its effect on one or more of the symptoms of PD.
Timing of administering each drug appropriately is crucial for the best control of symptoms.
Timing is first based on the expected onset and duration of action of each medication.

Each medication is given when it is expected to provide the best control of a symptom.
Each medication has its own potential side effects that may or may not appear in a specific patient.
Control of side effects is often achieved by dose/timing changes.

The health care professional must establish a clear picture of how well each drug controls PD symptoms over the day and must identify any side effects and when in the day they appear.

Help the patient maintain an accurate schedule of medications at all times.
Help the patient record and track side effects in his/her calendars/diaries.

KNOW THE MEDICATIONS AND DAILY DOSING SCHEDULE → DESCRIBE THE SYMPTOM CONTROL OVER THE DAY

KNOW THE SIDE EFFECTS OF EACH MEDICATION → ESTABLISH THE DAILY PATTERN OF SIDE EFFECTS

All changes in medication management should be based on facts derived from comparing the daily pattern of symptoms, the daily schedule of medications, and the daily record of side effects.

The best medication management of PD requires balancing the dose and timing of medications with the control of symptoms and the prevention/limitation of side effects.

A patient's therapeutic response to any medication may change over time and good management depends on regular visits and frequent communication between the medical team, the patient, and the caregiver.

Medication Management of Individuals With Parkinson's Disease

A common language . . .

Familiarize yourself with the following commonly used terms and phrases related to the experiences of Parkinson's disease patients:

"On" – The time period when medication is providing control of, or a decrease in, Parkinson's disease symptoms.

"Off" – The time period when medication has worn off and symptoms of Parkinson's disease have returned.

Wearing off – The time period between "on" and "off" when a patient senses that the medication is starting to lose effectiveness and that symptoms are beginning to return.

Dyskinesia(s) – Involuntary movements that may occur in the face, limbs, neck, and trunk indicating that too much dopamine is available in the brain at that time.

Dystonia(s) – Muscle tightness or cramping that may be accompanied by pain.

Tremor – Rhythmic shaking or trembling movements, fast or slow, that usually occur at rest and generally affect the extremities.

Medication Management of Individuals With Parkinson's Disease (Continued)

Symptoms experienced by Parkinson's disease patients:

An individual will usually not experience all symptoms; symptoms will vary from person to person.

Primary	**Secondary**		
–Rigidity (muscle stiffness)	–Handwriting difficulties	–Orthostatic hypotension	–Anxiety
–Bradykinesia (slowness of movements)	–Changes in facial expression	–Fatigue	–Depression
–Tremor	–Changes in bowel/bladder function	–Sleep disturbance	–Dysautonomia
–Postural instability (impaired balance)	–Speech/swallowing difficulties	–Sexual dysfunction	

Potential Complications of Therapy

–Motor fluctuations	–Dyskinesia (involuntary movement)	–Confusion/psychosis
–Wearing off	–Behavioral changes	–Sleep disturbance
–"On-Off"	–Hallucinations	–orthostatic hypotension

Special Considerations:

-Differentiate between *tremor* (a Parkinson's disease symptom) and *dyskinesia* (a medication side effect).

-Make every effort to administer medications on time (the *patient's* time).

-Note that stress, sleep deprivation, infection, dehydration, and changes in other coexisting diseases can affect an individual's response to medications.

Medications Used for Parkinson's Disease

Carbidopa/Levodopa

The primary drug used to relieve Parkinson's symptoms is a combination of carbidopa and levodopa. In the brain, levodopa is converted to dopamine, the neurotransmitter that is deficient in Parkinson's disease. Carbidopa allows levodopa to enter the brain with fewer side effects than levodopa alone. The dose is written as a fraction with the top number representing the mg (amount) of carbidopa, and the bottom number representing the mg (amount) of levodopa.

Side Effects: As with most medications, side effects may occur when treatment starts, when the dose is changed, or at any time during treatment; not everyone may experience side effects. Potential side effects include: nausea, hypotension, dyskinesia, confusion, hallucinations, dystonias, wearing-off effect, "on-off" effect, sleepiness, insomnia, dry mouth, skin rash.

Special Considerations: Never abruptly stop carbidopa/levodopa without consulting the health care prescriber.
Since carbidopa/levodopa is taken at frequent intervals during the day, patients often use special wristwatches or pillboxes with multiple alarm settings; these are available at many department stores and pharmacies.

Sinemet® (carbidopa/levodopa)	**Sinemet CR®** (CR = Controlled-release or long-acting form)	**Parcopa®** (A form that will dissolve in the mouth)
Available as: 10/100, 25/100, 25/250	Available as: 25/100, 50/200	Available as: 10/100, 25/100, 25/250
Dosing issues: Tablet is scored—partially cut—so that the tablet may be easily broken in half. Take 1/2 hour to 1 hour before meals or 2 hours after meals. Take with an entire glass of water or juice.	Dosing issues: NEVER chew, crush, or cut the controlled-release/long-acting form (CR). Take with an entire glass of water or juice.	Dosing issues: Can be taken with/without fluid/drink.

Medications Used for Parkinson's Disease (Continued)

Dopamine Agonists

These drugs mimic the effects of dopamine by stimulating dopamine receptors directly. They are most commonly used in combination with carbidopa/levodopa when additional help is needed to control Parkinson's symptoms and to smooth out the fluctuations of mobility that occur over time. Dopamine agonists may also be used as initial therapy to delay the need for carbidopa/levodopa.

Side Effects: See individual medication(s).

Special Considerations: Changes in dose (increases and decreases) are made slowly; achieving the best dose may take several weeks.
Dizziness, light-headedness, or headache may indicate medication-related hypotension; evaluate via supine/standing BP measurements over several days.
Evaluate/discuss any baseline levels of compulsive behaviors (e.g., gambling, hypersexuality) as these behaviors may occur.
Potential safety concerns with sudden onset of sleep during activities, including driving, reported with some dopamine agonist use.

Pramipexole dihydrochloride (Mirapex®)	**Ropinirole (Requip® Requip LA®)**	**Rotigotine (Neupro®) Transdermal patch**	**Bromocriptine mesylate (Parlodel®)**	**Apomorphine (Apokyn®)**
Available as: .125 mg, .25 mg, .5 mg, 1.0 mg, 1.5 mg	.25 mg,. 5 mg, 1, 2, 3, 4, 5 mg Long acting 2, 4, 8 mg	Available as: 2 mg, 4 mg, 6 mg patch	Available as: 2.5 mg tablet 5 mg capsule	Injectable formulation, available in a pen-type injector (SC = under the skin)
Side Effects: Nausea, postural hypotension, hallucinations, constipation, insomnia, somnolence, dyskinesia, dystonia, compulsive behaviors.	Side Effects: Nausea, hypotension, somnolence, headache, vomiting, dyskinesia, hallucinations, compulsive behaviors.	Side Effects: Skin reactions at patch site, postural hypotension, nausea, vomiting, hallucinations, somnolence, insomnia, applied every 24 hours.	Side Effects: Postural hypotension, nausea, confusion, hallucinations, dystonia, ergotism, headache.	Primarily used to treat acute "off" periods. Requires specific/detailed training.
				Contraindicated in patients allergic to sulfites or if treated with 5HT3 antagonists such as ondansetron, granisetron, etc.

Please refer to drug reference guides for dose ranges and a complete list of adverse effects.

<table>
<tr>
<td colspan="2">COMT Inhibitors
These medications block catechol-O-methyltransferase, an enzyme that breaks down dopamine. This action increases the availability of dopamine. COMT Inhibitors must be used in combination with carbidopa/levodopa in order to be effective.
Side Effects: See individual medications.
Special Considerations: Individuals with a history of liver disease should not use these drugs.</td>
<td colspan="2">Carbidopa/levodopa/entacapone (Stalevo®)
Tablets containing:
mg cabidopa/# mg levodopa/ # mg entacapone
Available Doses:
Stalevo 50: 12.5 mg/50 mg/200 mg
Stalevo 100: 25 mg/100 mg/200 mg
Stalevo 150: 37.5 mg/150 mg/200 mg
Stalevo 200: 50 mg/200 mg/200 mg</td>
</tr>
<tr>
<td>Tolcapone (Tasmar®)
Available doses: Tablet, 100 mg, 200 mg.
Side Effects: Diarrhea, dyskinesia, hypotension, hallucinations, nausea, urine discoloration.</td>
<td>Side Effects: Darkened saliva or urine, diarrhea, fatigue, dizziness, abdominal pain, dyskinesia, pain, constipation, hallucinations.</td>
<td rowspan="2">Entacapone (Comtan®)
Available doses: Tablet 200 mg
Side Effects: Diarrhea, dyskinesia, hypotension, hallucinations, nausea, urine discoloration.</td>
<td rowspan="2">Special Considerations: Comtan does not require monitoring of liver function.</td>
</tr>
<tr>
<td>Special Considerations: The FDA warns that Tasmar should be used as an adjunct only in PD patients on carbidopa/levodopa who are experiencing symptom fluctuation and who are not responding to, or are not appropriate candidates for, other therapies.
Tasmar requires liver monitoring due to an increased risk of liver toxicity.</td>
<td>Special Considerations:
See carbidopa/levodopa and Comtan (entacapone)</td>
</tr>
</table>

Medications Used for Parkinson's Disease (Continued)

MAO type-B Inhibitors – These drugs decrease the breakdown of dopamine. They are used in combination with Sinemet or as a first-time therapy to relieve symptoms of Parkinson's disease.

Side Effects: Excessive dopamine symptoms, gastrointestinal upset (insomnia with selegiline).

Special Considerations: Should **not** be taken with Demerol (meperidine). Patients scheduled for elective surgery should notify their health care provider so that the medication is discontinued or appropriate measures are taken.

Cautious use with certain SSRIs to avoid risk of confusion.

Last dose should be taken no later than 2 P.M. (risk of insomnia).

Selegiline 5 mg tablets (Eldepryl®)	**Orally disintegrating selegiline (Zelapar©)**	**Rasagiline (Azilect® Tablets 1 mg, 2 mg)**
Available as: 5 mg tablets	**Available as:** 1.25 mg tablets **Special Considerations:** Instruct the patient to let the medication absorb under the tongue. Patient should not eat or drink anything for 5 minutes after medication intake to fully absorb the medication.	**Available as:** 0.5 mg and 1.0 mg tablets **Special Considerations:** A low tyramine diet is recommended; medications such as omeprazole and ciprofloxacin may alter the potency of the medication; try to avoid mixing with cold medications that contain pseudoephedrine.

<table>
<tr><td colspan="2">Anticholinergics
These drugs are primarily used to treat tremor early in the course of treatment. They help maintain a proper balance of brain chemicals acetylcholine and dopamine.
Side Effects: Dry mouth, blurred vision, urinary retention, confusion, hallucinations, sedation, constipation, vomiting, loss of appetite, weight loss, listlessness, nervousness.
Special Considerations: Persons with glaucoma should not use this medication. The side effects of confusion or difficulty urinating may necessitate halting the use of this medication.</td><td colspan="2">Amantadine (Symmetrel®)
Amantadine is an antiviral compound believed to boost the release of dopamine in the brain.
Side Effects: Swelling of ankles and legs, "Livido reticularis," hallucinations, confusion.
Special Considerations:
Amantadine should be used cautiously in patients who have heart and/or renal failure.
Available doses: Capsules 100 mg, liquid syrup</td></tr>
<tr><td>Benztropine mesylate (Cogentin®)
Available doses: Tablets 0.5 mg, 1.0 mg, 2.0 mg</td><td>Biperiden hydrochloride (Akineton®)
Available doses: Tablets 2 mg</td><td>Procyclidine hydrochloride (Kemadrin®):
Available doses: Tablets 5 mg</td><td>Trihexyphenidyl HCL (Artane®)
Available doses: Tablets 2.0 mg, 5.0 mg</td></tr>
</table>

Please refer to drug reference guides for dose ranges and a complete list of adverse effects.

Appendix IV
Additional Notes

MEDICATION SCHEDULE

Patient: ____________________ Effective Date: ___ / ___ / ___

Neurologist: _______________

(Times)

Medications:	Dose:	-----	-----	-----	-----	------	------	------	------	-----

ADDITIONAL INSTRUCTIONS:

*Please call with any questions or concerns

NOTES

Index